"A clogged system has to flush out the goo so it can continue to work as efficiently as possible. And my system needed a kick-start and clean-up crew. When Lisa started working on me, I could feel my mind starting to reconnect to my tired body. My sinuses started to drain. I felt hope again. I noticed a hum of life back with me after she coaxed my lymphatic system into a more receptive state. It felt wonderful and I only question why we don't all use these techniques on a regular basis to keep our bodies and minds humming smoothly. I'll be reading this book with my son so he will grow with awareness of his body, how to clean house (so to speak) and help it do what it can do so miraculously. I am so grateful Lisa is sharing her wisdom and techniques with us. Truly a life-changing and enhancing method."

—Selma Blair, Actress

"Lymphatic massage is an incredibly therapeutic technique for optimizing a person's health, improving his or her immune system, and decreasing inflammation. I find that lymphatic massage is not celebrated enough in the Western medical world in regards to preventive health and of course treating states of disease and imbalance. Lisa Levitt Gainsley is a gifted, trusted, and passionate certified lymphedema specialist. Her book is an invaluable resource—we would all benefit from her wisdom and experience. I, for one, know that I would be very excited to share this book with my patients and colleagues!"

—Rachel Frankenthal, PA-C, MPH, Gynecologic Oncology at David Geffen
School of Medicine, UCLA

"Once you have experienced Lisa Gainsley's healing hands it will be hard to not want to experience that for a lifetime. Lisa's deep knowledge about the body's essential detoxification pathway and immune system booster, the often ignored lymphatic system, has been a big game changer in my life. And the best part is, I see the results of her massage treatments immediately. And now with this well-detailed book, I am beyond thrilled for the world to get a dose of Lisa's kind and gentle but powerful and life-changing knowledge and be equipped to try some of it out on their own bodies."

—Freida Pinto, Actress

"This book of Lisa's is the culmination of a lifetime devoted to improving people's lives. I was fortunate enough to be one of those people."

—Larry David, Actor and Producer

"Lisa is the most trusted voice in lymphatic health. Her method helps me feel great, gives me more energy, and keeps me glowing. Now everyone can enjoy instant results from her easy-to-follow self-massage tips. This book is an invaluable resource everyone should keep in their holistic first aid kit."

—Candace Nelson, Entrepreneur, Sprinkles Cupcakes

"In the last few years I have been drawn as part of my healing and self-care to learn more about my body and with that came a deeper understanding of my lymphatic system. It's such an integral part of our bodies yet no one really tells you about it and how it works. Through my discoveries I was fortunate enough to meet Lisa, who changed everything for me and taught me most of what I know about my lymph and how important it is to staying healthy, removing toxins, and looking and feeling good. She is truly an expert in this field and has a very gentle and holistic approach. Through seeing Lisa for treatments she taught me hands-on techniques I could do myself on a daily basis, which for me has been a game changer in the way I feel but also in the way I connect to my body."

—Jenni Kayne, Entrepreneur, Jenni Kayne Lifestyle

"Lisa Levitt Gainsley is an expert in the field of lymphatic therapy. Lisa has been helping people thrive after cancer treatment for over twenty years. The facts of how lymph controls health is knowledge known by the medical community that Lisa makes accessible in her book. Her expertise in teaching people how to maintain a properly functioning lymph system is invaluable. Lisa's method of lymphatic self-massage is one of the most impactful and easy tools in a person's health arsenal. Her book is an essential guide to boost immunity that I recommend to anyone whether they are facing an illness or looking for concrete ways to enjoy vibrant health."

—Gottfried E. Konecny, M.D., Professor of Medicine, and
Obstetrics and Gynecology, UCLA

THE

BOOK

OF

LYMPH

THE
BOOK
OF
LYMPH

Self-Care Practices
to Enhance
Immunity, Health,
and Beauty

LISA LEVITT GAINSLEY, CLT

ILLUSTRATIONS BY EMMA LYDDON

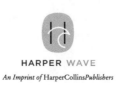

HARPER WAVE

An Imprint of HarperCollins*Publishers*

This book contains advice and information relating to health care. It should be used to supplement rather than replace the advice of your doctor or another trained health professional. If you know or suspect you have a health problem, or have recently undergone surgery, it is recommended that you seek your physician's advice before embarking on any medical program or treatment. All efforts have been made to assure the accuracy of the information contained in this book as of the date of publication. This publisher and the author disclaim liability for any medical outcomes that may occur as a result of applying the methods suggested in this book.

Names and identifying characteristics of individuals have been changed to preserve their privacy.

FIRST EDITION

Designed by Bonni Leon-Berman

Library of Congress Cataloging-in-Publication Data

Names: Gainsley, Lisa Levitt, author.
Title: The book of lymph : self-care practices to enhance immunity, health, and beauty / Lisa Levitt Gainsley.
Description: First edition. | New York, NY : Harper Wave, 2021. | Includes index. |
Identifiers: LCCN 2020051624 (print) | LCCN 2020051625 (ebook) |
ISBN 9780063049130 (hardback) | ISBN 9780063049154 (epub)
Subjects: LCSH: Lymphatics—Massage. | Massage therapy.
Classification: LCC RM723.L96 G25 2021 (print) | LCC RM723.L96 (ebook) |
DDC 615.8/22—dc23
LC record available at https://lccn.loc.gov/2020051624
LC ebook record available at https://lccn.loc.gov/2020051625

23 24 25 26 TC 10 9 8 7 6 5

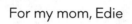
For my mom, Edie

CONTENTS

INTRODUCTION

A flower blossoms thanks to the nutrient-rich environment in which it's born. We relish its smell and its beauty even when the real glory belongs to its network of roots.

Within each of us there exists a similar invisible system that is continually working beneath the surface and is connected to every inch of our body—tidying up and sending vitality and support to ensure that we are the most radiant and healthiest version of ourselves. This is the lymphatic system.

Lymph constantly replenishes us. Every cell in your body is literally bathed by its fluid; it's the often overlooked missing link to vibrant health. Your lymphatic system cleanses and nourishes every other system of your body. It acts like a garbage collector, sweeping immune cells through your body to weed out anything that threatens your well-being, making lymph your first line of defense against illness. Your lymphatic system is responsible for maintaining your fluid balance, which can help keep inflammation—an underlying factor in many diseases—at bay. It enables you to properly digest and eliminate food. It's also what gives your skin its healthy glow.

Harnessing the power of lymph for self-healing has been my mission in life. I've dedicated my entire career to working with people's lymphatic systems because the results are nothing short of life changing. I've worked with thousands of people who've come to me for help with nearly every medical condition under the moon, from cancer to chronic fatigue, from gastrointestinal disorders to Lyme disease, eczema, acne, chronic headaches, and PMS. I've also treated many healthy young people who are interested in experiencing the detoxifying and beauty-enhancing effects of lymphatic drainage while seeking to avoid the chronic illnesses their parents deal with.

Often my clients have struggled to locate someone who offers the treatments I do; it's not easy to find a qualified lymphatic therapist. They don't exist in every town or community. Some practitioners are trained solely in the beauty benefits of lymphatic massage, while others have certifications to work with more serious health issues and enhance the immune systems of their clients. I wish it were easier for everyone to access a lymphatic expert, but what I've learned over decades of experience is that although a qualified and experienced practitioner is a wonderful resource, everyone can learn the tools necessary to stimulate and strengthen their own lymphatic system. You can take an active role in self-healing with your own hands.

Maybe you've heard that you can stimulate your lymphatic system by rebounding on a trampoline, by dry-brushing, or by doing inversions in a yoga class, all of which are in fact ways to get your lymph flowing. The methods I will share with you in this book are even more efficient than any of these activities because they specifically target the areas where your immune cells do their most productive work—in your **lymph nodes.** You will learn simple, three-to-five-minute lymphatic self-massage sequences that will address your most pressing concerns, from focusing on immune health to aiding digestion to reducing bloat and achieving glowing skin. Unlike deep-tissue body work—what most people think of when they hear the word "massage"—lymphatic therapy is much gentler. Lymphatic massage strokes concentrate on the fluid found just under the skin, which is why the touch is so light and nurturing.

How can manipulating lymph offer so many benefits? When lymph flows, everything else flows, too. Lymphatic self-massage helps eliminate toxic materials, and when you do it on a regular basis, you prevent toxins from accumulating and damaging your body's systems. The routines I offer in this book are grounded in science, tested and perfected over my decades of clinical work, and almost as relaxing as a day at the spa. Once you apply these routines consistently, they will become as routine as brushing your teeth. Not only will you love how you feel, but you'll tap into your body's innate ability to cleanse itself from the inside out. You'll also find that the practice of self-massage can improve your mood and lift your emotions as well as mitigate physical ailments such as headaches, earaches, and fluid retention. Lymphatic self-massage will soon become your favorite tool in your holistic toolbox. It will enable you to release congestion in your body, reconnect to the flow of life, and enjoy luminous health.

MY JOURNEY TO LYMPHATIC HEALTH

I've spent my entire adult life learning and practicing the healing tradition of lymphatic massage. My path began in the late 1970s, the moment my parents sat my brother and me down on the brown plaid couch in our living room and told us that our mother had cancer. I was just shy of eleven years old.

Before I knew it, I was immersed in all aspects of her illness. First there were the sterile hospitals and the waiting rooms of brain surgeons, assimilating words such as *radiation* and *chemotherapy* and their consequences into my schoolgirl vocabulary. Then there was the realm of alternative healing practices that was of equal importance to my family. This included the Silva Method, aimed at healing oneself by entering a deeper state of consciousness through meditation. Different from other types of meditation I would later study, the Silva Method uses guided visualization techniques to improve well-being. My brother and I would carve out forts and comfy places for ourselves on the floor and meditate, imagining laboratories and healing sanctuaries inspired by the ocean, the moon, and grassy hillsides, *willing* our mom to get better. It was in these visions that I took my first forays into the idea of healing.

I used to lie with my mother while she listened to cassette tapes of tranquil waters with blooming lily ponds and meditate, my hand on her body. We ate carob and kefir, probiotics and macrobiotics, fermented veggies and spirulina—all wildly fringe choices at the time. The comforting smell of herbal teas and potted plants in our home provided a cozy antithesis to the stark and painful procedures my mother endured. This kind of healing seemed so normal and logical that I never thought of it as unusual.

I knew that those moments with my mother were sacred. They were special and tender. I wasn't afraid of her illness. For someone that young, I felt remarkably calm and stable. Looking back at it all now, I see that I was developing sensitivity. In those years I learned how to touch someone who was fragile. I enjoyed being helpful and seeing how much better my mom felt as a result of my touch.

When self-healing is an act of unconditional love, grace flows willingly. I had no idea how much that era would shape the trajectory of my life. After my mother's death, when I was thirteen, I looked for ways to make sense of her loss. I searched for meaning at the metaphysical bookstore the Bodhi Tree in Los Angeles. I was drawn to books on reincarnation, Hinduism, Buddhism, and existentialism on the wooden shelves. I spent hours roaming up and down the aisles, hanging on to quotes about varying cultures' views on death and the meaning of life. I started a yoga practice. The void within me pushed me to experiment with how I felt in my body, and I became driven by the desire to pursue what preventive health practices could mean and how to achieve them.

By the time I attended college at San Francisco State University, I was sensitive to how my body felt in various environments, how my mood changed around certain friends and under stress, and the effect the foods I ate had on my belly. I took courses in holistic health and yoga and became obsessed with anthropology, the mind/body connection, and, in particular, the way different cultures approached healing. It was the late 1980s and early 1990s, and alternative modes of healing weren't yet widely accepted in Western medicine. (Acupuncture, for example, was seen as woo-woo then; now it is used in practically every pain clinic and hospital in the country.) I graduated with a degree in cultural anthropology and a minor in religious studies, my intention being to study ancient healing traditions and integrate them to help people get well. But I realized I wanted a more hands-on and less academically oriented career.

When I enrolled in the Institute of Conscious BodyWork, a massage school set among the redwood trees of Northern California, I was immediately drawn to the practice of manual lymphatic drainage massage. Over the next five years, I completed my studies to become a certified massage therapist, with an emphasis on the lymphatic system. I loved the way lymphatic massage felt; I'd never experienced anything like it before. The rhythm and cadence of the strokes felt as soothing as undulating ocean waves. Time and time again I was transported to how I had felt in my body before my mom's death—that sense of "home in myself" without the existence of trauma. After multiple sessions, my chronic digestive issues improved, my bloating reduced, and my acne went away. The more I studied the intricate patterns of the lymph system and how the particular series of strokes of lymphatic massage are grounded in science and physiology, the more passionate I became. I learned the direct connection between the lymphatic system, the immune system, and the digestive system, and also that lymphatic massage has a calming effect on the nervous system. One of my teachers taught us tai chi and qigong so that the rhythm of our lymphatic massage strokes would be akin to a moving meditation. Finally, when I realized that lymphatic massage could benefit cancer patients, I knew I had found my life's work. My career is a love story to the memory of my mother. Her memory is what guides my devotion to helping others.

Two decades ago, when I was working as a Certified Lymphedema Therapist at UCLA Medical Center, most of my clients were cancer patients whose treatments had caused a disease of their lymph system. Although chemotherapy, radiation, and surgery save lives, the treatments can also create a lesser-known condition called **lymphedema**, chronic swelling of a body part, for which there is still no cure. When your lymph is in a diseased state, your body can't effectively remove toxins and bacteria, leading to swelling in an arm or leg or chronic inflammation in the abdomen and face. My training afforded me the ability to help those patients manage their condition. What I also found was that after treatments, the skin on my clients' faces had a healthy, hydrated glow, whereas an hour before it had looked ashen and gray. Week after week, my clients marveled at how much better they felt in their joints, how their numbness and tingling symptoms subsided. The heaviness in their limbs went away. They lost weight. And after so many constipating medical treatments, they were finally able to go to the bathroom! "It's the first time I felt human since the diagnosis," they'd say.

The question that kept coming to me in those years was "Why aren't we working *earlier* to improve people's lymphatic systems *before* there's a problem?" Certainly one reason was that insurance wasn't going to pay for it. In California, my clients were accustomed to paying out of pocket for deep-tissue massages, facials, laser hair removal, and other luxuries to improve their appearance. Meanwhile, I knew that the benefits of lymphatic treatments were twofold: they enhanced the appearance of the skin and slimmed the waistline, and they bolstered patients' health at the cellular level. Lymphatic massage addresses the root cause of chronic conditions, not just their symptoms. By having their congested toxins swept out, patients got more bang for their buck: immune-boosting benefits with glowing results.

When I left UCLA and opened my own practice in 2001, none of my colleagues were working *preventively*. A majority of my business was still working with cancer patients, but the word quickly got out that people were finding relief from long-standing health issues. I saw clients with eczema, chronic fatigue, sinusitis, acne, constipation, lupus, Lyme disease, even amyotrophic lateral sclerosis (ALS, also known as Lou Gehrig's disease). With my lymphatic massage technique, I was having huge success in a multitude of applications in a short amount of time. Since my training had prepared me to understand the systemic flow of lymph, I began to develop specific sequences targeted to address any ailment that walked through my door. Few people knew that lymphatic drainage had actually been created to target symptoms such as the common cold and inflammation—which was why my clients were amazed with the results. Before I knew it, I had more requests for appointments than I could manage.

This book is the result of the time I spent in between sessions fielding a dizzying array of requests from my patients about how they could maintain their lymphatic health (and their radiant results). Before I knew it, I was developing materials to meet the needs only lymphatic *self-massage* could address, and I began to show my clients how to do simple self-massage sequences. What we all noticed was profound: whether I was the one performing the sequences or my clients were practicing on their own, the results were undeniable. Those who took my advice (doing three-to-five-minute self-massage sequences daily) reported experiencing less inflammation, better digestion, fewer PMS symptoms, and fewer headaches. They slept better and got fewer colds, and their stress levels improved. Their skin was lustrous, and their wrinkles relaxed. Some of my clients who were at an increased risk of developing breast cancer even showed a decrease in breast density on their mammograms.

That's when I knew I needed to write a guide to lymphatic care—not just for my clients but for everyone, so they could replicate my hands-on sessions at home. What most excites me about this book is its potential to benefit the health of each and every reader. Whether you're looking to improve your skin or your immune system, balance your hormones, or level your moods, this book will serve all your needs. It's a lot of power in one simple package.

Today lymphatic drainage has gone from a little-known niche to one of the most discussed buzzwords in wellness. In my practice I've seen lymphatic drainage provide the following benefits:

Accelerate: Weight loss, healing from illness, athletic injuries, and postsurgical recovery

Achieve: Glowing skin

Balance: Immunity

Flush: Toxins

Improve: Digestion, earaches, energy, healing, and sleep

Reduce: Anxiety and nervous system disorders; bloating; cancer treatment side effects; cellulite; cold and flu symptoms; eczema; headaches; lymphedema symptoms; mental fog; pre- and postnatal symptoms; sore throats; symptoms of autoimmune diseases and conditions such as Crohn's disease, chronic fatigue syndrome, fibromyalgia, Graves' disease, Lyme disease, and lupus; and thyroid issues

Relieve: Constipation, menstrual cramps, and perimenopausal and menopausal symptoms

Treat: Inflammation

I realize that this list may seem too good to be true, but I assure you that the benefits of lymphatic massage are very real—which is why it's increasingly recommended by a wide array of physicians, including oncologists and radiologists. They know that your lymphatic system connects every other bodily system; its effects on your health are wide-ranging because its physiological geography is expansive.

Our cells are constantly being renewed, creating opportunities for new healthy patterns to emerge. Lymphatic massage will connect the dots between your physical symptoms and your emotional well-being. When you cultivate the practice of lymphatic self-care, you will be addressing both at the same time. By attacking the root of the problem, you will clear out stress and undesirable symptoms. You will instantly look and feel refreshed after a lymphatic self-massage, not unlike the way you feel after taking a bath or a minivacation at a spa.

These pages will serve as a resource that you can turn to time and again as any unwanted symptoms arise. It's the full suite of my very best sequences, strategies, tips, and rituals that I teach in my workshops and perform on my clients every day.

Part I covers the basic science of the lymphatic system and why lymphatic self-massage is essential to maintaining your health.

Part II contains lymphatic self-massage sequences for radiant beauty, improved immunity, weight management, stress reduction, better sleep, and so much more. You will become empowered to improve your well-being and take control of how you look and feel. These lymph optimization strategies are quick, easy, and therapeutic. Soon you will be able to do self-massage anywhere you like, anytime you want. All you need is the soft touch of your own fingers. It's incredibly nourishing and soothing.

Part III is full of holistic remedies to complement your self-massage sequences. There's information on skin care, holistic treatments, and exercise, backed by scientific research on how they pertain to lymph. This section will show you how to get the most out of your self-care routines.

Of course, your health will fluctuate throughout your life, but your ability to support your own well-being is a constant. It is my hope that this book will empower you with tools to support you on your journey. When we do the things that make us feel *good*, we unlock the foundation of health.

Part I

THE POWER
AND SCIENCE
OF LYMPH

Chapter 1

RIVERS OF IMMUNITY

You're already exercising. You're eating healthfully. You're balancing stress (or trying to!). But you still don't feel great. I hear this every day in my practice. Clients come in with observations such as "Something doesn't feel right," "I'm tired all the time. I eat well, I sleep, I work out, I take supplements—but I have no energy," "I'm always constipated," and "I've tried *everything*, but I just feel out of sorts."

Until recently, medical practitioners typically paid little attention to these kinds of comments, in part, I believe, because they are vague enough not to be potentially lethal symptoms of a major illness—even while they diminish quality of life. These symptoms *are* telling us something; they *are* evidence of imbalances. In my practice, I treat these concerns not as unimportant complaints but as clues to how to restore health. When I address a patient's *lymphatic* health, such symptoms often abate, and my client experiences both physical and emotional improvements. This is because the lymphatic system is connected to every other system in the body—including the nervous system, the digestive system, and the neurological system—with branches that run through its wide geography like an intricate web of rivers. When it functions properly, you feel vibrant, energetic, and clear-headed. You're able to digest and eliminate the food you eat, sleep well at night, and focus on what you need to accomplish during the day. You don't get sick all the time, and you seem to breeze through cold and flu season.

When your lymphatic system is congested, on the other hand, you may feel lethargic and stuck. You may be constipated and headachey and experience more aches and pains than usual. It may seem as though you come down with a cold the instant anyone in your proximity sneezes. You might even be more anxious than usual for seemingly no reason. What you can't see is that underneath the surface of your skin, the flow of your lymph "rivers" has likely slowed to a crawl, inhibiting organ function across your body. From your liver to your skin to your brain, all of your organs rely on the lymphatic system for optimal functioning.

Tending to your lymphatic health is as important as your daily flossing and brushing ritual; we know that we remove bacteria and plaque from our teeth to maintain good dental hygiene. Maintaining lymphatic health is like that: if you don't tend to it consistently, problems can accumulate over time.

Think about how good you feel after cleaning your home, getting your car washed, or organizing your desk. Most people feel freer and lighter after such a cleanup. Once you've removed the grime, dispensed with the garbage, and tidied up your environment, new oxygen can flow through your space. Lymphatic self-massage does the same thing for you *internally*. It's like a cleaning or tidying up for your body. You will feel lighter and more energized in just five minutes because you will have reduced the stressors that are causing congestion and stagnation. You will go from feeling stuck to being free flowing.

But before I teach you how to enjoy these benefits, let me walk you through the anatomy and function of your lymphatic system so you can better understand how it works and why it's such a powerful force in your well-being.

BASICS OF THE LYMPHATIC SYSTEM

What is lymph, exactly, and why didn't you learn about it in school when you were taught about your circulatory and digestive systems? Given how essential the lymphatic system is to your immune health, it's staggering to me that most of us were taught virtually nothing about it! So let's start with the basics.

There are two circulatory systems in your body:

Your cardiovascular system, which consists of your heart and your blood vessels. Your heart is at the center of this system, and its network distributes blood throughout the body. The blood vessels transport oxygen and nutrients to cells. Your arteries carry blood away from your heart, and your veins carry it back in a continuous loop through your cells, removing carbon dioxide and delivering vital nutrients that keep you alive and regulate your body temperature.

Your lymphatic system, considered to be your "second" circulatory system, is the sanitation and recycling system of your body. Just as you have two sets of pipes in your home—one set that brings in fresh water and another that removes dirty water—your lymphatic system is the bonus set of plumbing that filters and removes excess waste from your body. It's approximately twice as vast as the cardiovascular system, but it doesn't have a central pump like the heart to move the fluid around. Lymph flows in only one direction: toward your heart. Because it is not propelled by a master pump, its flow relies on the pulsing of nearby arteries, skeletal muscle contractions, and breathing. That's why self-massage, breath work, and exercise are invaluable to good lymphatic health.

Your lymphatic system plays a number of critical roles in your body. It's an essential part of the immune system, producing white blood cells with the power to destroy harmful pathogens. It acts as a garbage collector, filtering out bacteria and toxins that can cause disease. It aids the digestive system by absorbing fat and fatty acids from your gut and transporting them back to your bloodstream, making them available as fuel to your cells. And finally, it maintains the fluid balance in your body by collecting, purifying, and draining excess fluids so your tissues don't swell. We'll explore all of these valuable roles in more detail shortly, but first, let's take a closer look at the intricate geography of the lymphatic system.

THE ANATOMY OF THE LYMPHATIC SYSTEM

Throughout your life, your lymphatic system continuously distributes immune cells across your body. When you look at the map of where your lymph flows, lymph nodes appear like gas stations along the highway of their vessel network. Lymph nodes are where the white blood cells called lymphocytes do their job of eliminating pathogens and harmful substances from the **interstitial fluid**—the fluid space between your cells— before it continues on its way to its final destination in the bloodstream.

The way lymph circulates through the body is in no way random; it is carefully mapped out. **Lymphatic fluid** moves inward from your extremities toward your heart. If you've studied geology, you know that rivers and streams collect water from one area and direct it toward a greater outlet such as an ocean. Your body is no different; your own pathways move lymphatic fluid like rivers, first to clusters of lymph nodes, then ultimately to your greater outlet: your bloodstream. Understanding these currents of the lymphatic system is critical to understanding why a lymphatic drainage massage is different from a typical deep-tissue massage. This will lay the foundation for cultivating your self-massage practice.

THE ATLAS OF LYMPH

When I see clients for the first time, I always show them this illustration. Most people have no idea that lymphatic vessels run through their entire body in a similar way to their blood vessels. Notice their systemic nature, the linked chain of vessels, capillaries, and ducts that run through nearly every inch of your body. The lymphatic system is an intricate network of vessels, capillaries, precollectors, collectors, and trunks that transport fluids from surrounding cells to lymph nodes. The nodes act as filtering stations, where white blood cells called **macrophages** and **lymphocytes** engulf and destroy harmful material before returning the fluid to the bloodstream, where it is eventually processed through the kidneys and liver and eliminated via bowel movements and urination.

Lymph is formed from the waste fluid of your body's cells. Each day, fluid seeps out of your blood capillaries and into the interstitial fluid. Although some of it is reabsorbed by blood capillaries, the job of your lymphatic system is to collect the remaining fluid (also referred to as the **lymph load**), which is made up

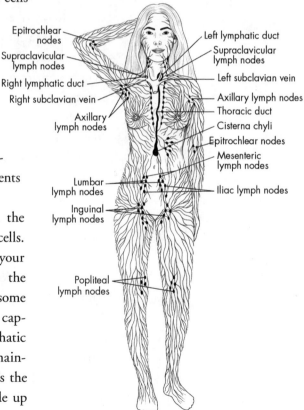

Epitrochlear nodes

Supraclavicular lymph nodes

Right lymphatic duct

Right subclavian vein

Axillary lymph nodes

Lumbar lymph nodes

Inguinal lymph nodes

Popliteal lymph nodes

Left lymphatic duct

Supraclavicular lymph nodes

Left subclavian vein

Axillary lymph nodes

Thoracic duct

Cisterna chyli

Epitrochlear nodes

Mesenteric lymph nodes

Iliac lymph nodes

of waste that's too big for your blood capillaries to absorb—including metabolic waste, proteins, hormones, fat-soluble vitamins, and immune cells—in order to prevent an accumulation of toxic debris in your tissues. That fluid enters the lymphatic system through tiny **lymphatic capillaries** shaped like fingers, located just underneath the top layer of your skin. Lymphatic capillaries are present all through your body, including in your digestive tract, reproductive system, and respiratory system. They have overlapping cells that open and close to absorb fluid, similarly to

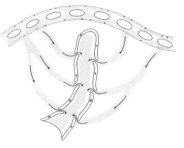

sponges or the way a plant's root system draws water into itself. They are also permeable, which allows tissue fluid, bacteria, viruses, and cancer cells to enter the system for purification.

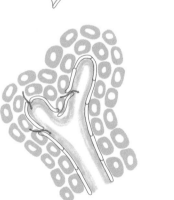

Lymphatic fluid is made up of approximately 50 percent nutrient-rich plasma proteins (plasma leaves the body's cells after it has delivered its nutrients) as well as harmful invaders that your venous system isn't able to re-collect. After the lymphatic fluid has been absorbed by the spongy capillaries, it travels through a series of one-way superficial lymphatic vessels toward the areas in your body where lymph nodes are located for purification. Your body transports approximately three liters (that's six pints) of cleansed lymphatic fluid back into your bloodstream daily to start its journey all over again.

The way the lymphatic system captures the body's cellular debris from your blood vessels is similar to the way rain gutters collect leaves and particles and rainfall runoff. If a gutter doesn't work properly, germ-laden trash gets clogged up in it and then overflows in a heaping mess that ends up strewn all over your lawn.

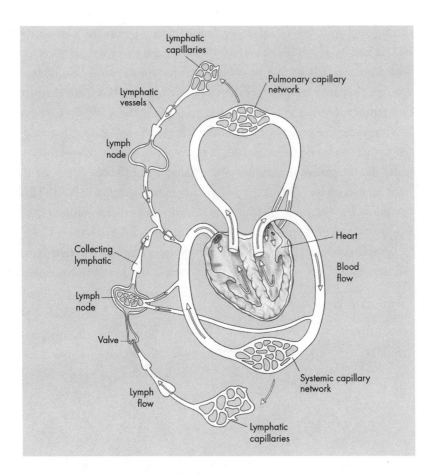

Lymphatic capillaries

Pulmonary capillary network

Lymphatic vessels

Lymph node

Collecting lymphatic

Heart

Blood flow

Lymph node

Valve

Lymph flow

Systemic capillary network

Lymphatic capillaries

LYMPH NODES

Your lymph nodes are the cornerstone of lymphatic massage. In the sequences in part II, you'll learn how to massage the nodes, found in most **hinges**, or joints that allow movement in one direction, of your body: your head, neck, armpits, sternum, abdomen, the crease at the top of your thighs, your elbow creases, and behind your knees.

You have anywhere from five hundred to eight hundred lymph nodes throughout your body, typically grouped around veins in adipose, or fat, tissues. Your lymph nodes are where bacteria and viruses meet up with immune cells so that your body can mount a critical immune response. They may be no larger than a pea or a kidney bean, but they are constantly surveying your insides for nefarious activity. When they are healthy, their size varies from 2 millimeters to 2.5 centimeters in diameter. Lymph nodes don't regenerate, so if any are surgically removed (typically due to cancer treatment), a mechanical insufficiency can result, impairing your body's ability to eliminate excess lymphatic fluid. This can put you at risk of developing lymphedema and other disorders of the lymphatic system (I will discuss these conditions in detail in part II).

Lymphatic fluid is brought into the lymph nodes by **afferent lymphatic vessels**. There, macrophages get to work, straining bacteria out of

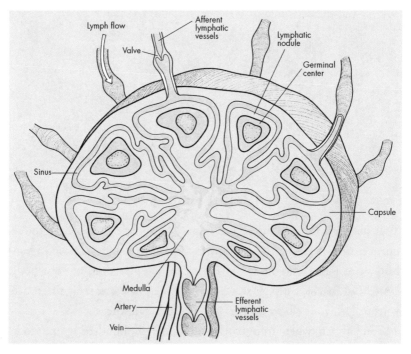

the lymph. Then lymphocytes engulf and destroy other material they recognize as harmful. Lymphatic fluid can go through several lymph nodes before it's fully cleaned out. Certain substances that cannot be wiped out (such as coals, dusts, and dyes) are stored in the node indefinitely.

Once the fluid has gone through this process, it reaches the **efferent lymphatic vessels**, which transport lymphatic fluid out of the nodes through a complex, one-way network of vessels and valves toward your heart, from which it is recirculated back into your bloodstream, toxin free. This is why lymph is sometimes referred to as "the great recycler": It does for your body what you do for the environment when you place your household recycling out on the curb, allowing it to be transported to a processing plant, where it's sterilized and repurposed.

Many people first learn about their lymph nodes when they're fighting an infection and the nodes swell up with the large amount of white blood cells needed to combat the germs. Maybe you've experienced this when you've come down with a cold; your lymph nodes (usually those in your neck) became enlarged and possibly even painful to the touch. Although you don't want to massage yourself when you have an active infection, knowing the **atlas of lymph** and how to self-massage properly will help accelerate healing and alleviate uncomfortable symptoms in your body.

The Language of Lymph

Learning about lymph and self-massage can be a bit like visiting a new city for the first time. It's exciting, but it can also feel overwhelming. Before you skip ahead to the massage sequences, it's important to consult a map and better orient yourself to your new surroundings.

I like to use scientific terms as much as possible whenever I teach anyone about lymph. I don't learn languages easily, so I've included a

Glossary of Lymph Terms on page 318 so you can refer to it as much as you need to. I believe it's important to learn the proper scientific terminology, as it will enable you to have informed conversations with your doctors and practitioners about anything going on in your body.

Also, as you'll see throughout this book, I strongly believe in the power of imagery. Words and intentions can help us heal. If you've ever taken yoga, remember how hard it was to learn and say the Sanskrit names of all those poses? But after only a few sessions, I bet those asanas seemed as though they had always been a part of your vernacular. I promise you, lymphatic terms will be rolling off your tongue in no time!

LAYERS OF LYMPH

Similarly to an onion, your lymphatic system has layers: the superficial layer and the deeper network. I tell my clients that understanding this basic concept will help them get the best results from their self-care practices.

The **superficial lymphatic layer** is located in the dermis, just under your epidermis, or the outermost layer of skin. As you know, your skin provides a barrier against foreign substances and is one way you eliminate toxins, through your sweat. The majority of your superficial lymphatic vessels, including capillaries and other lymph collectors, exist above the muscle bed. The vast lymphatic network exists here alongside your blood capillaries. Particles that escape from these capillaries move into the interstitial fluid, where they then become part of the lymphatic system. *This is where your hands will be accessing most of your lymph in your self-massage sequences.*

The **deeper lymphatic network** drains organs and deeper regions of your body. These regions of your body include **trunks and ducts**. Trunks are formed from collecting vessels that unite to drain large areas of the body after lymphatic fluid has been filtered in the lymph nodes. The convergence of many efferent lymphatic vessels delivers fluid to the right lymphatic duct (responsible for draining one-quarter of the lymphatic fluid) and the left lymphatic duct (which drains the remaining three-quarters of fluid), which comes from the body's largest lymphatic vessel, the **thoracic duct**.

The thoracic duct, which runs from your abdomen up the front of your body to the left subclavian vein, delivers your purified lymph back into your bloodstream. The right and left subclavian veins enter the venous system at its junction with the internal jugular vein near the clavicle.

Usually, superficial lymphatic vessels follow the same routes as veins, and deeper lymphatic vessels follow the same routes as arteries. The deep network is also responsible for taking fats from your gut and the fluid from your lower limbs. It can be stimulated by deep diaphragmatic breathing. This is one of the reasons why breath work is so valuable during all of your self-massage sequences: it activates deep lymph circulation.

A well-functioning lymphatic system provides the transportation for your immune system; it's one of the vital highways of your body. If either of the two layers of lymphatic pathways is congested or malfunctioning (due to hereditary factors, lymph node removal, or other stressors), cellular waste and proteins can accumulate in your tissues.

Lymph also regulates your body's fluid balance and is one reason you feel lighter and brighter after a lymphatic treatment and why your face and abdomen appear less puffy and bloated. Every day, when small protein molecules leak out of your blood capillary walls, they increase the osmotic pressure of your interstitial fluid. What this means is that fluid accumulates in the tissue spaces due to the limited return of fluid back into your blood capillaries. If this process continues unchecked, your blood volume and blood pressure decrease significantly while the volume of your tissue fluid increases. The result is swelling, or **edema.**

This is where lymphatic capillaries play such an important role: they are the entry point into the lymphatic network, where excess interstitial fluid and protein molecules are absorbed that will ultimately return to the bloodstream to manage your body's fluid balance. Focusing lymphatic massage on the **superficial fluid layer**—using direction-specific strokes to flush out toxins—while tending to the **deeper lymph structures** with your breathing and abdominal massage mimics your body's ability to circulate protective immune cells and restore your good health. That's why self-massage sequences work so well: they target the movement and filtration rate of lymph.

As I mentioned, unlike your main circulatory system, which is powered by your heart, lymph doesn't have a central pump. But lymph *does*

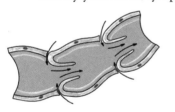 have its own unique process to circulate its way through your body; it's propelled by both *intrinsic* and *extrinsic* means.

Lymphatic vessels have one-way valves called **lymphangions**. These are microscopic heart-shaped chains, like tiny pearls on necklaces, that fill up with lymphatic fluid. Smooth muscle contractions produce electrical impulses six to twelve times each minute that control the ceaseless opening and closing, contracting and relaxing, of your lymphangions. These contractions are an example of the *intrinsic* way your lymphatic fluid circulates, a process called **angiomotoricity.** The intrinsic pump relies on the spontaneous contractions of the muscle cells within the wall of the lymphangion.

The one-way valves of your lymphangions act like propellers preventing any backflow of lymphatic fluid. *Pressing too hard or too deeply during self-massage can cause these valves to spasm and suspend the movement of lymph.* This is one of the reasons why some people swell up in extreme heat—when they are in a sauna or steam room—or in extreme cold— like in an ice bath: the extreme temperature change on the surface of the skin can cause a temporary strain to lymph movement. Using a slow cadence when you are doing lymphatic massage will prevent the backflow of lymphatic fluid.

The second driving force of lymph circulation is *extrinsic*; your lymphatic system depends on blood vessel pulsations, heart contractions, skeletal muscle contractions, muscle contractions in the gastrointestinal tract, and breathing movements to generate the pressure that propels lymph. In part II, you will learn specific lymphatic massage strokes and breathing techniques to affect your lymph movement.

LYMPHOTOMES AND WATERSHEDS

Now that you understand the anatomy of lymph and how it moves around your body, let me introduce you to **lymphotomes**, the territories of your body that drain lymphatic fluid toward regional lymph nodes. Lymphotomes are part of the superficial layer that defines the direction of lymph flow during a massage. My clients rely on this illustration because it really helps them understand *where* they are going to massage themselves.

The locations of these drainage patterns are neatly organized by regions of your body—think of them as the "mapping" of drainage. The boundaries separating the lymphotomes are called **watersheds**. Lymphatic fluid is directed to specific clusters of lymph nodes. During your self-massage, you will work in specific directions toward the nodes that

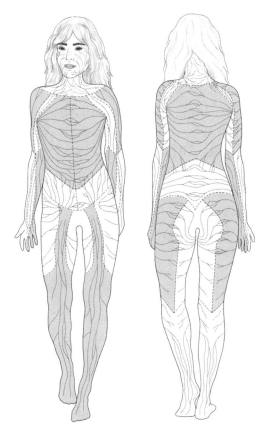

drain a particular section of your body. It's kind of like coloring within the outlines of a drawing; knowing the directions of lymphotomes is essential, as it will guide your practice.

We tend to think of drainage as something that flows downward, thanks to gravity. But that's not always how lymphatic drainage works. Understanding the mapping of where your lymph flows is crucial. For the purposes of your self-massage sequences, you'll be working with approximately six different lymphotomes. This will allow you to use the sequences in this book intuitively, confidently, and for maximum benefits.

Not only does lymph flow up the body, it also flows from the back of your body toward the front, toward the heart. This is why, in my practice, I always start my sessions with my clients lying faceup: I want to stimulate the lymph nodes in the front of the body before I do anything else.

After the lymphatic fluid in the lymphotomes is drained, a quarter of the lymph from the upper right quadrant of your body empties into your right lymphatic duct near your collarbone at the subclavian vein, where it enters your bloodstream. This includes your right arm, the right side of your chest, your right breast, the right side of your upper torso (front and back), and the right half of your head, neck, and face. The other three-quarters of the lymphatic fluid drains into the thoracic duct that empties into your left subclavian vein. That fluid comes from the lower half of your body—both of your legs and your abdomen—as well as the left side of your chest, your left breast, and the left side of your upper torso (front and back), and the left half of your head, neck, and face. These ducts join the large veins above your heart, where they return your filtered lymph back into the venous system.

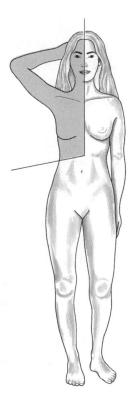

Like the earth, approximately 70 percent of our bodies is made up of water: this includes our blood, interstitial fluid, and lymph. The function of the nutrients and what surrounds them is moved and informed by our fluid layer. Our bodies need these fluids, which work together to protect and heal us daily. Whether the exchange of fluids in our bodies works well or not makes the vital difference in the health of our cells, our tissues, and the inner workings of our organs.

The three liters of lymph that circulate through your body every day have a **transport capacity**. The movement of lymph is slow, and it can become overwhelmed by too much congestion. I liken the concept of lymph load to a bus filled with people during rush hour. It's important that as many people exit the bus as get on at each stop so that the bus can run smoothly and efficiently. You'll know your lymphatic system is becoming overwhelmed when you feel the nodes in your neck swell up. That's an indication that waste is building up at a faster pace than you're able to get rid of it—as if too many people got onto a bus and not enough got off—and your body is fighting an increased level of toxins.

Another way I like to describe lymph transportation is through another traffic analogy: the dreaded bottleneck. If one exit on the freeway is closed, you end up with a backlog of cars with nowhere to go. When lymph nodes and pathways are congested with too much waste, or if lymph nodes have been removed, a bottleneck will occur somewhere along the lymph transportation line. And if your body can't keep eliminating waste, other bodily functions will suffer. Fortunately, with lymphatic self-massage and self-care techniques, you can use a detour to clear out stagnant waste. You can refer to the section on Lymphedema on page 237 for how to re-route lymph fluid if you've had surgery or lymph nodes removed.

The transport capacity of the lymphatic system is the maximum amount of lymphatic fluid that can be transported at a time; the lymphatic system doesn't function at maximum capacity all the time. The ability of the lymphatics to function well depends on lymph load and the ability of the system to transport it. If your lymphatic system needs to handle an increased load (such as an infection), typically it can deal with it due to what's called a **functional reserve**. The functional reserve will react to increased activity and additional volume of **lymph fluid** in order to get the fluid to where it needs to go. Fortunately, in a typical healthy person, the transport capacity is greater than the amount of lymph it's expected to transport. This gives your body an opportunity to deal with an excess load so it can regulate it sufficiently.

But if you push your lymphatic system too far, just like allowing more onto the bus than its allotted occupancy or not stopping to get gas or add oil when your car needs it, your system gets overburdened. When it does, the amount of lymphatic fluid that needs to be transported will exceed the maximum transport capacity. When that happens, the result is excess fluid accumulation in the interstitial space, which causes swelling. Sometimes the swelling is obvious enough that you'll be able to see or touch it. This is called a dynamic insufficiency of the lymphatic system. When the lymph collectors are working at maximum capacity over a long period of time (or if they've been damaged due to surgery or other traumas), they can get strained. If this continues for months, it can cause damage to the structure of the walls and valves of the lymphatic system, resulting in what's called mechanical insufficiency.

At this point, reducing the amount of lymphatic fluid as soon as possible is essential—and you can easily do this regularly by implementing the pillars of lymphatic health outlined later in this book. You can stimulate your lymphatic system with exercise, which will increase your lymphatic contraction rate approximately tenfold—but you can also move your lymph *even more efficiently* with the specific strokes you do during regular lymphatic self-massage. Why? Because you'll be working directly on your lymph nodes. In fact, this is one reason why lymphatic massage is unique among other massage techniques: it targets your immune system—*not* your muscles and tissues. In the next chapter I'll explain in more detail what happens when you have a dynamic and mechanical insufficiency of the lymphatic system and how they impact your health.

How Lymph Got Its Name

Lympha means "water" in Greek. It's the perfect word to illustrate the ancient beauty and mechanics of this system. Lymph is the fluid that bathes every cell and gives your body its innate ability to heal itself.

Closely associated with the word *nymph*—a spirit that preserved the rivers and springs for purification in ancient Greece—Lympha was also an ancient Roman agricultural deity embodying the divine aspects of water. The word was later used as a noun to represent a source of fresh water. That's why it's referred to as your lymphatic aquarium of health!

LYMPHATIC VASCULATURE:
A PEEK INSIDE THE VESSELS AND VALVES
THAT ARE KEEPING YOU HEALTHY

Lymphatic capillaries are larger than blood capillaries but still very small. Located just beneath the epidermis of your skin, they weave throughout the connective tissue, absorbing excess waste and proteins from interstitial fluid. These permeable capillaries contain overlapping endothelial cells, which are responsible for the release of enzymes that control vascular contraction and relaxation, blood clotting, immune function, and platelet bonding. When the surrounding interstitial pressure changes, these lymphatic vessels either expand and fill with lymph or contract and push lymph into **lymphatic precollectors**, which facilitate lymphatic fluid to then enter larger transporting vessels, known as **lymphatic collectors** and often referred to as lymphatic vessels. The collectors are oriented to absorb fluid. They have more structure than blood capillaries; they contain smooth muscle cells and valves that are instrumental in absorption and lymph movement. They regulate lymph flow one way.

The collectors direct lymph flow into your regional lymph nodes. These vessels have valves that prevent the backflow of fluid and maintain a distal-to-proximal transportation of fluid toward the lymph nodes. In other words, this is where your lymphatic system is propelled from your limbs and farthest regions of your body toward your heart.

The lymphatic collector segments are separated by heart-shaped valves that lie horizontally, which is the key to understanding your self-massage strokes. This is the layer you will access with your self-massage sequences. It's why in most cases you'll use your palms instead of your finger-tips—so you can mimic the horizontal action of these collectors. You will be working in this super-ficial layer to move lymphatic fluid toward your lymph nodes. When you stretch the walls of these collectors with lymphatic self-massage strokes and deep breathing, you increase the pulsation of the lymph collectors—which propels lymph!

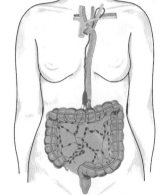

The thoracic duct is considered to be the main collecting vessel because it drains three-quarters of your lymph into your bloodstream. It begins in the abdomen at the **cisterna chyli**, the sac that absorbs fat from the small intestine, which gives lymph its milky white color, and moves fluid from the lower half of your body up to your heart. It runs alongside your spine, starting around your lumbar and thoracic vertebra (TL2 to T11), and is about 2 to 5 millimeters in diameter and varies from 36 to 45 centimeters long with a diameter of 1 to 5 millimeters.

There is a lot of variability in the structure of the thoracic duct, but its job is so invaluable that you will often see it mentioned in your self-

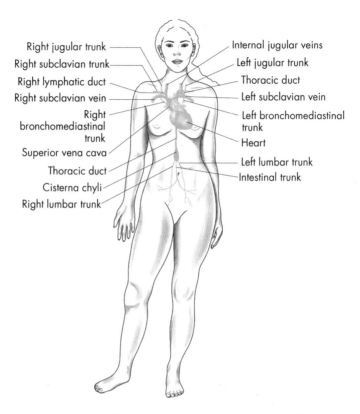

Right jugular trunk
Right subclavian trunk
Right lymphatic duct
Right subclavian vein
Right bronchomediastinal trunk
Superior vena cava
Thoracic duct
Cisterna chyli
Right lumbar trunk

Internal jugular veins
Left jugular trunk
Thoracic duct
Left subclavian vein
Left bronchomediastinal trunk
Heart
Left lumbar trunk
Intestinal trunk

massage sequences. Deep diaphragmatic breathing impacts the function of the thoracic duct. *This is why breath work is so important to good lymph flow.* When you breathe from your diaphragm, it stimulates lymph flow into the bloodstream.

Lymphatic trunks are deeper regions of the lymph network that receive lymphatic fluid that's already been passed through and cleaned out in the lymph nodes. Each trunk is named for the territory it drains, and is formed by a convergence of efferent vessels that empties lymph into either the thoracic duct or the right lymphatic duct where it enters your blood circulation.

LYMPH: YOUR UNSEEN PROTECTOR

Your lymphatic system is an integral part of your immune system; without it, your cardiovascular system would stop working and you couldn't live for more than a day or two!

As a fetus develops, stem cells that will become white blood cells and lymphocytes are formed in the bone marrow and migrate to **lymphoid organs** throughout your body—which you probably didn't realize are part of the lymphatic system and are needed to keep you healthy.

These lymphoid organs—your bone marrow, tonsils and adenoids, thymus, **mucosa-associated lymphoid tissue (MALT)**, **gut-associated lymphoid tissue (GALT)**, spleen, appendix, Peyer's patches, and urinary tract—are small masses of lymph tissue found where a lot of bacteria tends to accumulate, so they are close by in order to fight any infections. They are safeguards of your immune system and play an important part in your body's defense mechanism and its resistance to disease.

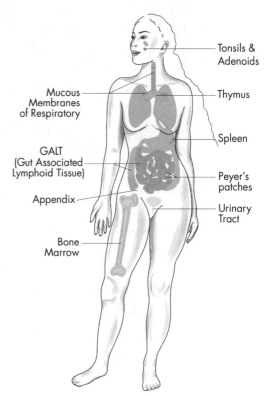

Fifty percent of lymphoid tissue falls under the umbrella term mucosa-associated lymphoid tissue (MALT), including the digestive, urinary, and respiratory tracts: it filters debris that is passed through your skin or the mucous membranes of your eyes, nose, and mouth and digestive tract, preventing pathogens from entering the mucous membrane lining and into the bodily fluids. Your tonsils and adenoids trap pathogens from the air you breathe in and the food you eat; your spleen filters blood, produces lymphocytes, and stores platelets and immune cells; and your thymus is where cancer-fighting T cells are matured. You also have lymph nodes in your gut that are often referred to as gut-associated lymphoid tissue (GALT), which includes the appendix, Peyer's patches (small masses of lymphoid tissue found primarily in the ilium of the small intestine), and some isolated lymphoid follicles (ILFs) in the small intestine.

GALT antigens launch an invaluable immune response to preserve equilibrium in your intestines. *In fact, the lymphatics in your gut make up approximately 70 percent of your immune system.* They are the first line of defense against food-borne illness. Millions of specialized lymphatic vessels located in the villi of your small intestine, called **lacteals**, are responsible for helping your body extract nutrients from the food you eat—absorbing fats, fat-soluble vitamins (lipids), electrolytes, and proteins and transporting them back to your bloodstream to be used as fuel. When lymph absorbs fat and lipids through a sac at the base of the thoracic duct (the cisterna chyli), its unique milky white color is created.

The lymphoid organs produce B and T lymphocytes, the white blood cells essential to fighting the infections you'll have over the course of your entire life. B cells make antibodies and are derived from bone marrow; T cells are matured in the thymus. In addition, after birth, lymphatic tissue accumulates in the appendix, where it helps to mature B lymphocytes and an antigen called immunoglobin A. Physicians used to think that the appendix was basically useless, but they know now that that notion was incorrect! Although the role of the appendix is greatly reduced as you age, it's essential in forming the molecules that will direct the movement of lymphocytes throughout the body.

The lymphatic system is part of both your innate and adaptive immune systems. "Innate immunity" immediately identifies and eliminates pathogens to prevent the spread of disease. Your lymphoid organs, natural killer cells, macrophages, leukocytes, dendritic cells, and other cells are part of it, since lymph serves as a pipeline for lymphocytes and immune cells to mingle and decipher what's harmful and what isn't.

"Adaptive immunity" (sometimes referred to as the "acquired immune system") is not an immediate but a long-term process. It uses fewer but more specific white blood cells, such as B and T lymphocytes, which identify and multiply to eliminate particular pathogens, mounting a substantial response against germs that the body recognizes as "nonself." Your body remembers this foreign matter so it can recognize it again if necessary. For example, when you get an illness like the measles, once you've recovered, your body has the ability to defend itself against the illness again, so you're now immune to it. Unfortunately, this is not true of all infectious illnesses. The tricky part of the adaptive response comes when the immune system going after the "nonself" makes an error and attacks itself—which can result in an autoimmune disorder such as lupus or rheumatoid arthritis.

It's essential that your body be able to pinpoint and defend itself against pathogens so you can maintain optimal health, and thereby lymphatic health. By providing you with the immune power to fight disease and expel toxins, lymph is literally the superhero of your immune system. You will start to notice that you can gauge where you stand on what's referred to as the lymphatic health continuum. When you have a balanced immune response, you are flowing easily on the continuum.

But there may be periods of your life when you get more frequent colds or chronic inflammation that causes lymphatic transport insufficiency, adversely affecting your immune system. The pendulum of health is influenced by many factors. Once you recognize the contribution lymph plays, you can utilize the pillars of lymphatic health to turn the tide. Every time you do any of the sequences in this book, you are improving your immune system. I can't think of a better argument for incorporating it into your daily life than these physiological facts. It's just common sense!

In the next chapter, you'll see how the rivers of lymph flow through and affect the health of every major system in your body. When one of them is out of harmony, you may experience a wide range of symptoms you may not even recognize as being related to your lymphatic health. Once you understand the interconnectedness of your lymph and organ function, you'll soon gain the tools to guide your own vessel along the waters within.

Lymph Through the Ages

When I introduce people to their lymphatic system, I like to start at the beginning. People have been curious about lymph for a very long time.

For centuries, many cultures—including those of India, Greece, Rome, Egypt, and China—made note of the lymphatic system. Their ancient texts refer to lymph nodes and lymphatic vessels as meridians, **rajas**, and **dathus**; Hippocrates, the "Father of Medicine" (ca. 460–ca. 370 BC) called the lymphatic fluid "white blood," and referred to it as "phlegmatic temperament," one of his four temperaments (the other three being sanguine temperament, choleric temperament, and melancholic temperament). Another ancient Greek physician by the name of Herophilos (ca. 335–ca. 280 BC) wrote that he had found "vessels emerging from the intestine enter a number of gland-like bodies," as well as lymph nodes and "milky veins"—the lymphatic system!

But those civilizations couldn't distinguish between lymph and blood, most likely because they lacked the tools to see that lymph has its own unique and extensive vascular network. Since it is microscopic, the entire network of lymph that travels through the body was too tiny to have been detected in those days.

Research on medicine and anatomy was discouraged during the Middle Ages, so it wasn't until the Renaissance that classical learning and exploration into the body came back into vogue. The seventeenth century was the golden age for investigation of the lymphatic system. Around 1622, the Italian physician and surgeon Gaspare Aselli made the first differentiation between lymphatic vessels, veins, and gut lacteals (lymph vessels in the small intestine that absorb dietary fat). Many people attribute the discovery of the lymphatic system to him. In 1637, a Dane, Thomas Bartholin, described the lymphatic system as "a process that purifies the body and regulates irrigation, swelling, and edema." He called the vessels "vasa lymphatica" and their content "lymph."

Olof Rudbeck, a Swedish scientist (1630–1708), was the first anatomist who recognized and understood the lymphatic system and its circulation as a completely intermingled system in the human body. In 1647, the Frenchman Jean Pacquet's breakthroughs included demonstrating that abdominal lymph nodes channel lymphatic fluid from the cisterna chyli up the thoracic duct and into lymph nodes in the subclavian vein at the neck before recirculating the lymph back into the blood circulation. By 1692, mercury injections proved to be the first means of how to see lymph flow. Fast-forward nearly two hundred years to 1885, when a Frenchman, Marie Philibert Constant Sappey, made a huge atlas of the lymphatic system—one that we still use.

In the late 1800s, several doctors treated elephantiasis as a chronic condition of the lymphatic system using massage, skin care, and exercises. The Austrian-Belgian surgeon Alexander von Winiwarter (1848–1917) was one of the first physicians who used manual lymphatic drainage techniques in hospitals combined with exercise, compression, skin care, and hygiene, which laid the foundation for future treatment for lymphedema patients.

In 1922, an American doctor of osteopathy, Frederick Millard, coined the term *lymphatic drainage* with the first hands-on technique and published *Applied Anatomy of the Lymphatics*. And in 1937, an Australian pathologist named Howard Florey (who later played a role in developing penicillin) was able to show that the lymphatic nodes enlarge during inflammation.

It wasn't until the 1930s that the Danish massage practitioner Dr. Emil Vodder and his wife, Estrid, who developed the "manual lymphatic drainage method," coined the term *lymphology* while they were working as physiotherapists in France. Many of their patients came for help after damp European winters left them with swollen lymph nodes and sinus problems thanks to frequent colds and flu. Using extensive clinical experience, they compiled systematic massage movements to facilitate draining lymph pathways slowly, rhythmically, and with an extremely light touch. The Vodders discovered that their method consistently cleared tissue stagnation and aided immunity. They taught manual lymphatic drainage for decades, and their system became the basis of my training. In 1993, Drs. Michael and Ethel Földi published *Das Lymphödem und verwandte Krankheiten: Vorbeugung und Behandlung* (Lymphoedema, Methods of Treatment and Control) in Germany; they are credited with developing the gold standard for lymphedema care known as **Complete Decongestive Therapy (CDT)** and still maintain one of the world's leading clinics for lymphedema therapy.

Lymph through the Ages

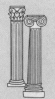

460 - 280 B.C.

Ancient cultures and physcians, by the likes of Hippocrates and Herophilos, refer to the lymph system as nodes, vessels, milky veins, meridians, rajas and dathus, white blood and lymphatic temperament

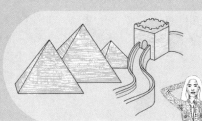

1622

Gasparo Asselli makes the first differentiation between lymphatic vessels, veins, and gut lacteals

1630 - 1708

Olef Rudbeck discovers the lymph systems's circulation as completely intermingled

1637

Dane Thomas Bartholine discovers that the lymphatic system regulates irrigation, swelling and edema; he names the vessels' content "lymph"

1647

Jean Pacquet understands the lymph system is circulated through the cisterna chyli and thoracic duct

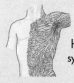

1885

Phillip Sappey makes a huge atlas of the lymphatic system that is still used today

1848 - 1910

Alexander Winiwarter discovers manual lymphatic drainage techniques for lymphedema, such as compression

1920s - 1930s

Frederic Millard coins the term "Lymphatic Drainage"; Howard Florey discovers that lymph nodes enlarge during inflammation; the Vodders develop the manual lymphatic drainage method coined "lymphology"

1993

"Lymphoedema, Methods of Treatment and Control," is published by Michael and Ethel Foeldi

Chapter 2

YOUR MISSING LINK TO HEALTH

The power of your lymphatic system is truly formidable. Not only is it at the center of your body's ability to identify and defend against many common diseases, but researchers have also identified the potential of the lymphatic system to play a leading role in fighting illnesses that have long confounded the medical community. In fact, in a talk given by one of the directors of the National Institutes of Health (NIH) to the LE&RN organization in March 2019, it was stated that studying the lymphatic system may lead to unlocking a cure for Alzheimer's, infectious disease, gastrointestinal disorders, and more. In other words, they anticipate that further insight into the function of the lymphatic system will yield groundbreaking discoveries. Although it took some time for the medical establishment to fully understand the breadth and significance of the lymphatic system, it's now a fast-growing field of scientific inquiry. What a truly exciting time to be in the field of lymphatic health!

It's significant that scientists at the NIH recognize that the influence of our lymphatic system may be broader than we now realize. You receive millions of messages from your body every day—from your senses to your emotions to physical symptoms such as aches and pains. All of these messages are valuable; they provide critical information about what's going on deep within your cells. Some of this information can be addressed easily with a little caretaking: you might blend up a green smoothie if you're running low on energy, make an appointment with your therapist if you're feeling down, or take a warm bath at the end of a tiring workday. Other signals, even ones that may seem relatively minor, such as chronic headaches, continual back pain, or unexplained weight loss, are serious warnings to pay attention to a specific aspect of your health. In this chapter, we'll take a closer look at the known ways in which lymph connects with other bodily systems. As you'll soon come to realize, lymph is the vital river that regulates homeostasis in every corner of your being.

LYMPHATIC CONGESTION

As you learned in the previous chapter, your lymphatic network is a slow-moving system that propels fluid through all its vessels approximately six to twelve times per minute. If you have excess debris in your tissues, your lymphatic system may become even more sluggish. When your lymph load and transport capacity are overwhelmed—what I refer to as lymphatic congestion—problematic health issues can arise.

Symptoms of improper lymph flow may be triggered by a physiological or stressful emotional event. You may suffer from bloating, aches and pains, intermittent digestive troubles, and persistent fatigue—discomforts that are immediately apparent. Other symptoms such as eczema, chronic constipation, and weight gain can creep up over time to snowball into problems that you may not realize pertain to your lymphatic system. In addition, stress hormones such as cortisol and adrenaline, which are chronically released due to anxiety and stressful situations, can exacerbate any physiological symptoms you may already have. Your physical health impacts your mental health, and vice versa.

As I'll discuss in chapter 5, physical exercise is an effective way to improve your lymphatic health as well as your mood, thanks in large part to the increase in lymphatic circulation and the release of endorphins that banish the effects of stress hormones. Remember, skeletal muscle contraction moves lymph. If you aren't exercising regularly, your body is less able to move toxic matter out of your tissues.

Lymph issues can manifest in a wide array of symptoms, and if you're anything like my clients, you've experienced at least a few of them at some point or another. Though it's true that many of these symptoms can have various causes, most people don't suspect that they have an underlying issue with their lymphatic health until they come to see me. In reality, poor lymph flow is a potent contributing factor that can alter where you stand on the lymphatic health continuum.

Signs of Lymphatic Congestion

Acne and skin breakouts
Allergies
Bloating and water retention
Blood clots
Brain fog
Bronchitis
Chemical pollutants
Chronic earaches/clogged ears
Constipation
Cuts slow to heal
Dehydration
Difficulty losing weight
Digestive issues
Edema
Enlarged lymph nodes
Fatigue
Fibroids/cysts
Headaches
Hormone imbalances, including
    cortisol, PMS, perimenopause,
    menopause
Inflamed tonsils
Itchy skin/eczema/rashes
Kidney disease
Lymphedema
Muscle stiffness/joint pain/arthritis
Obesity
Pain or discomfort while exercising
Puffiness in face and neck
Scar tissue
Sinus congestion and infections
Sore throats

Signs of Lymphatic Congestion

Stress   Upper respiratory issues
Swelling of joints; swelling of
  extremities on airplanes

RISK FACTORS FOR POOR
LYMPHATIC HEALTH

Some people experience symptoms due to risk factors that are out of their control. Risk factors may be inherited or acquired. For instance, you might be more susceptible to lymphatic overwhelm if you had surgery; if you underwent a cesarean section when you gave birth, the incision may have cut through superficial vessels that impede lymph flow, explaining why there is swelling near your scar. Or, as you'll see on page 129, if you have been exposed to environmental toxins, your lymphatic system may become overwhelmed by the toxic load in your body.

Genetic risk factors can result in an underdeveloped or misdeveloped lymphatic system. If you've noticed that one of your parents or grandparents or even an aunt has chronic swollen ankles; if you developed thick legs at puberty, as an adult, or during pregnancy; or if you've always had chronic inflammation in your limbs that doesn't subside, even with changes in your diet, you could have a genetic condition called primary lymphedema. Another genetic factor is having a gene called MTHFR, which interferes with the body's ability to detoxify sufficiently.

If you have any of these risk factors, I recommend regular lymphatic self-massage and a reevaluation of your diet and nutrition plan. You may also benefit from wearing **compression garments** such as socks, leggings, or sleeves to manage swelling in your extremities. They are especially useful in mitigating chronic inflammation as they create external pressure on the interstitial fluid that acts as a propellant for lymph flow. Use the applicable sequences in chapter 4 to assist your current condition.

Surgery of any kind, especially cancer treatment, lymph node removal, and radiation; elective surgeries such as face-lifts and rhinoplasty; and hip and knee replacements can impair lymph flow. Although lymphatic congestion is common among the general population, it impacts at least 30 to 40 percent of cancer patients more severely. Cancer patients who have had a disruption in their lymphatic system due to surgery, lymph node removal, lumpectomies, or radiation are at risk of developing a medical condition called **lymphedema**. Over time, the damage to the lymphatic system can be so great that extremities or limbs may swell with leaky interstitial fluid, leaving them vulnerable to immune compromise and a host of infections, including cellulitis.

If you have had surgery, including cancer surgery, I recommend turning to the "Athletic Injuries, Pre- and Postoperative Recovery, and Scar Tissue" and "Lymphedema" sequences beginning on page 232. Beginning your self-massage treatments prior to surgery is recommended to help mitigate the proliferation of lymphedema. If you are at risk of developing or have lymphedema, find a Certified Lymphedema Therapist to work with who can help you manage this condition. (For more information on how to locate a qualified practitioner, see page 317.)

Exposure to toxins can overload the lymphatic transport system. Scientists studying environmental toxicology are learning more about the effects of various toxins on our cells, as the alteration or hindrance of normal cellular activity can lead to inflammation, autoimmune disorders, and even cancer. Some of the most dangerous offenders are asbestos, environmental pollutants, mercury, mold, pesticides and herbicides, and some ingredients in household cleaning and skin care products.

To minimize your exposure to toxins, I recommend removing all household and skin care products that contain dangerous ingredients (such as carpet and upholstery cleansers containing PERC; cleansers containing solvents such as 2-butoxyethanol; window and other cleaners containing irritating ammonia and/or chlorine; oven cleaners containing sodium hydroxide; and formaldehyde in hair-straightening products, eyelash glue, and nail polish) and choosing organic food as often as possible. Although some toxins, such as coals and tattoo ink, can't be eliminated fully from the lymph nodes, you can continue to flush out other elements such as heavy metals resulting from your exposure to the environment (such as lead paint in older homes) or the foods you ingest (such as mercury in contaminated tuna) and the symptoms they create when they accumulate in the soft tissues of your body. You can find sequences that will help common symptoms of toxin buildup, such as those for headaches, earaches, and mental clarity in chapter 4. Also, the list of Lymphatic Holistic Remedies in chapter 5 provides information on how to detox regularly.

Taking certain medications, though necessary, can contribute to swelling in the body. If you have an underlying lymphatic mechanical insufficiency, some prescriptions may exacerbate a chronic issue. Be aware of this for any medications that include edema as a side effect, as diuretics can lead to fluid retention and increased protein retention in the interstitium; some diabetes meds can lead to sodium retention and congestive heart failure; and amantadine, an antiviral commonly used for Parkinson's disease, lists swelling in the hands, feet, or legs as a side effect.

If you take medications that cause swelling, speak with your doctor. I'm not suggesting that you stop taking your meds, but you should know that inflammation may be coming from places you might not expect.

As more research proves the integral role of lymph in finding treatments for various diseases, you can see that the lymphatic system is the missing link: better lymphatic flow equals better health.

Limb Swelling on an Airplane

Anna, a healthy, vibrant Italian mother in her forties who frequently flew to California on business trips, attended one of my workshops in search of relief from her persistently swollen legs. She'd struggled with swelling in her legs ever since she had gone through puberty, and during the long international flights she made regularly, her legs would swell so badly that she had difficulty putting on her shoes.

I explained that the discomfort and heavy, achy feeling in her extremities were classic symptoms of lymphatic congestion. Because the cabin pressure on planes is lower than on the ground, it can change the tissue pressure in your limbs, which is what helps propel lymph. If your body is absorbing less fluid into your lymphatic system, excess lymphatic fluid remains in the extracellular spaces and contributes to swelling. Low cabin pressure can also keep your blood from moving as quickly as it normally would. And since you're usually sitting still for hours on flights, the lack of muscle contractions can impede lymph and blood from circulating properly.

The easiest solution to flight-caused swelling is to wear compression socks, which give your limbs the extra external pressure they need to keep your lymph circulating properly, and to wear sneakers, which help compress your feet. In addition, doing the "Achy Limbs: Legs" sequence (page 223) before and after you fly will provide immediate relief. I also recommend getting up and moving around during the flight as much as you can, staying hydrated, and avoiding alcohol, caffeine, and salty foods, which cause you to retain water. If you are at risk of developing deep-vein thrombosis—aka blood clots—make sure you check with your physician if the swelling persists for several days after the flight.

THE LINK BETWEEN LYMPHATIC CONGESTION AND INFLAMMATION

Before we go further, it's crucial to clarify the term "inflammation," which is used a lot in wellness circles because it's at the root of so many disorders in the body. Inflammation shows that your body's immune defenses have been triggered in response to a toxic invader or injury. Many different immune system cells can come into play, and your lymphatic system is a critically important component, because your lymphatic vessels serve as a main transport route for the unwanted inflammatory cells to get into the lymph nodes, where your invader-fighting white blood cells can mount an immune response. But if your lymphatic vessels aren't functioning properly, their role in regulating that response will be inadequate. If your lymphatic vessels aren't as able to work at their usual pace, the lymph load may outweigh the transport capacity of the lymphatic system, causing a buildup of lymphatic fluid.

In addition, your lymphatic system regulates fluid homeostasis, because it's responsible for the drainage of excess fluid in your body. If left unchecked, excess fluid that comes from leaky, swollen blood vessels can lead to chronic inflammation in your tissues. With lymphatic self-massage, you will increase the transportation rate of lymphatic fluid, which can then help remove excess fluid and reduce inflammation in your body.

Edema and Lymphedema: What's the Difference?

It's easy to get confused about the difference between edema and lymphedema. The important distinction is that edema, or swelling categorized by low protein levels in interstitial fluid, can occur even when your lymphatic system is intact and functioning properly. Edema can be the result of capillary leakage in the interstitium or failure of the lymphatic system to return fluid to the bloodstream. It's the result of a high-output failure, meaning that the lymph load exceeds the transport capacity of the lymphatic system; this is referred to as dynamic insufficiency. The types of disorders in this category are chronic heart failure, chronic venous obstruction, deep-vein thrombosis, excess chronic inflammation, and tumors that obstruct venous return.

Lymphedema, on the other hand, happens when the transport capacity is disrupted, and the lymphatic system is damaged or malformed. It's a low-output failure that's recognizable by higher levels of protein in the interstitial fluid. As mentioned on page 19, it's referred to as mechanical insufficiency of the lymphatic system. This can happen due to genetics or as a result of scarring from surgery and/or radiation, blunt trauma, valvular insufficiencies, thrombosis, and obstruction of lymphatic vessels by tumors, lymph node removal, or surgery.

"Combined insufficiency" occurs when you have both a dynamic and mechanic insufficiency. The lymphatic system is impaired, the transport mechanism is reduced, and the lymph load is higher than what can be carried away. An example is when someone was born with a misdeveloped lymphatic system (primary congenital lymphedema) and develops a chronic venous insufficiency; a person's system has a combined disorder in which the transport capacity is reduced *and* the lymph load is increased.

ACUTE AND CHRONIC INFLAMMATION

Not all inflammation is bad. Acute inflammation is your body's response to a sudden injury to repair damaged tissue: smaller blood vessels dilate to allow more blood to reach the area, which results in swelling, redness, and heat. Then the white blood cells swoop in to make sure that no toxic invaders, such as bacteria that can enter the bloodstream when you have an open wound, cause further problems.

This is where your lymphatic system enters the picture to work with your blood circulation to heal the injured site; your body forms new blood (a process called angiogenesis) and lymphatic vessels (lymphangiogenesis) to simultaneously coordinate a response. While your blood cells do their jobs, your lymphatic system is circulating the immune cells to drain the injury site of excess cellular fluid and bacteria in the tissues, which is what reduces the levels of the pro-inflammatory cells that can cause even more swelling.

Acute inflammation subsides as the injury heals. This can be a pretty quick process if you've simply banged your shin or a lengthier process if you've broken a bone or gotten a cut that needed stitches to close. Chronic, prolonged inflammation, on the other hand, is a far more serious and potentially life-altering issue. It's not a specific disease or illness; it's a mechanical response within your body that occurs when acute inflammation persists. That means it's no longer a healing response but much more insidious. Low-level chronic inflammation plays a role in nearly every Western illness. According to the World Health Organization, chronic inflammatory diseases—including allergies and asthma, Alzheimer's disease, arthritis and other joint diseases, cardiovascular diseases, chronic obstructive pulmonary disease, and diabetes—today make up one of the greatest threats to human health.

One of the biggest problems with chronic inflammation is that it can be caused by so many different factors; often it's hard to know what triggered it, which makes it difficult to treat. Another problem is that it often unfolds silently, deep within your body. Standard lab tests don't always detect it; inflammation is typically diagnosed only with more sophisticated testing or in conjunction with the diagnosis of another medical condition, so it can take some time before you realize that it's causing problems. Inflammation can result from infections, exposure to toxins, autoimmune disorders, cellular defects, and recurrent episodes of acute inflammation. Some symptoms of inflammation include excess weight in particular spots, frequent infections, constant aches and pains, fatigue, mood disorders, and gastrointestinal issues. The risk factors are sometimes within your control (eating a healthy diet, avoiding smoking and exposure to other toxins, sleeping well, managing your stress levels), and sometimes they aren't (your age, genetic history, and hormone levels all play a role).

During acute inflammation, when the blood vessels expand (this is called vasodilation), the first type of white blood cells that arrive are short-lived neutrophils, followed by macrophages, lymphocytes, and plasma cells, which identify and destroy dangerous pathogens. But when something in the usual healing process goes haywire—and scientists still can't pinpoint an exact reason much of the time—cells don't heal properly. Instead, they are infiltrated by growth factors, enzymes, and cell-signaling protein molecules called cytokines that normally regulate your immune system response. You want cytokines to aid in the attack on the pathogens in your body, but they can also suddenly proliferate to kick your immune system into overdrive—what's called a cytokine storm. It's often mentioned in relation to the Spanish flu pandemic of 1918, SARS, or COVID-19, in which victims' cytokine storms cause rapid cell disintegration, particularly in the lungs, leading to permanent damage to tissues and an increased risk of death.

Chronic inflammation is also dangerous because it can create a cesspool of bacteria-laden stagnant fluid in your tissues. If unchecked, stagnant fluid becomes ripe for harboring a systemic infection like cellulitis, and your immune system becomes very stressed as it tries to fight it off. In other words, chronic inflammation can trigger your body to attack its own tissues, leading to a vicious cycle in which your immune system fights back, triggering even more inflammation and interfering with your lymphatic vessel function. This impedes your body's ability to remove toxins and regulate fluid balance, and your lymphatic system becomes congested.

Being able to rid your body of stagnant, congested lymph is exactly why lymphatic drainage massage is so helpful. The strokes you'll do to increase lymphatic vessel actions are designed to increase lymphatic circulation to eliminate pathogens and mitigate inflammation. Research shows that when lymphatic vessels are stimulated, there is a higher absorption rate of the inflammation-causing stagnant fluid, leading to a reduction in skin inflammation, arthritis, and weight loss, as well as a decreased severity of irritable bowel disease, including Crohn's disease and colitis. Take note of the "Signs of Lymphatic Congestion" on page 34; if you have several of them and they persist, you might be at risk of developing chronic inflammation. The more proactive you are in working with your lymphatic system, the quicker you can change undesirable patterns and improve your health.

When MDs Call on Lymphatic Drainage Specialists

Lymphatic therapists often collaborate with physicians across special-ties. One of my referrals came from an oncologist whose patient, in her late seventies, had developed lymphedema. She'd endured six surger-ies, including the removal of fifteen lymph nodes under her armpit, and she was experiencing swelling in her arm as a side effect of her many treatments.

When I first started seeing her, she complained of a heavy, achy, numb arm that was clearly swollen and much bigger than her other arm. She couldn't get the sleeve of her shirt to fit over her arm. Her range of motion was impacted, and she was depressed about her appearance. She was also getting sick a lot; her frequent colds were the result of her weakened immune system and accumulation of lymphatic fluid. Over the course of six months, I performed manual lymphatic drain-age, had her fit for compression garments, and I taught her lymphatic self-massage sequences she could do at home.

One day I received a call from the oncologist who had referred this patient to me. He called to express his gratitude for my work; not only was her arm less swollen, but her psychoemotional state had improved, too. Many people don't realize that a swollen, disfigured limb can also have as negative an effect on a person's emotional health as a cancer diagnosis has. Finally, my client was happy. She was hopeful. "You made a huge difference in the life of this woman. Not only does her arm look better, but she feels great, too! You made my job a whole lot easier," the doctor said. The next time I saw my client, she beamed as she showed off how she could fit into her favorite long-sleeved shirt. Then she gave me a big hug and said, "Thank you for making me feel like myself again. I haven't been this happy since I was told I was cancer free."

THE INTERCONNECTEDNESS OF
YOUR BODILY SYSTEMS

Your lymphatic system is one of eleven organ systems in your body. The others are the cardiovascular, digestive, endocrine, integumentary, muscular, nervous, reproductive, respiratory, skeletal, and urinary systems.

They all work together, of course, to keep you alive. And lymph is a crucial component of nutrient and hormone absorption, fluid homeostasis, and immune function.

So let's take a look at how your lymphatic system interacts with your digestive system (your gut and other digestive organs), your nervous system (the cognitive/neurological and emotional aspects of your brain), and your respiratory system (the way you breathe). I call this your gut/brain/lung/lymphatic connection.

LYMPHATIC HEALTH = DIGESTIVE HEALTH

Your gut is often referred to as your "second brain." Thanks to recent breakthroughs in the study of the microbiome—the collection of microorganisms found in your gastrointestinal tract—gut health has gone from a niche topic nutritionists and functional medical doctors lecture about to a topic of casual dinner conversation. We all have an enormous number of microorganisms in our GI tracts—more than 100 trillion. Many of these microbes support our health, especially as lymph fluid is drained by the **mesenteric lymph nodes** in your abdomen. The mesenteric lymph nodes determine if the nutrients and microbial substances that have entered the lymph fluid in the intestinal mucous membrane contain pathogens that must be destroyed. They play a critical role in food tolerance and serve as a line of defense to prevent systemic spread of microorganisms.

When the balance between beneficial and potentially harmful microbes is altered, your immune system suffers. You've experienced this if you've ever had gastrointestinal distress after taking antibiotics, which kills off both beneficial and harmful bacteria.

Your lymphatic system is an integral part of your digestive system, and it has two primary functions.

The first is to help with the processing of your food. Lymphatics are essential conduits for the absorption and transport of nutrients, hormones, some drugs, and other extracellular components from the digestive tract via the cisterna chyli and thoracic duct to your bloodstream.

Some fats and proteins are large molecules that are too big for your bloodstream to pick up and take to the cells where they can be utilized. Instead, it's up to your lymphatic system to transport fatty acids and lipids (in the form of chylomicrons in the intestines) to your liver, then back to your bloodstream from the thoracic duct. This is where those molecules turn into fuel, which improves your metabolism and your energy.

In addition, in the small intestine, lymph removes excess tissue waste and absorbs digested fat, also known as **chyle** (that's what turns the lymphatic fluid a milky white color), fatty acids, proteins,

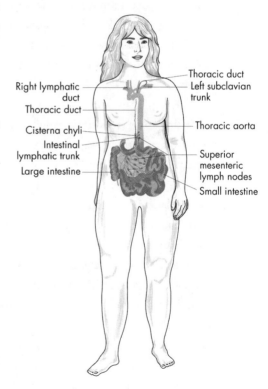

Right lymphatic duct
Thoracic duct
Cisterna chyli
Intestinal lymphatic trunk
Large intestine
Thoracic duct
Left subclavian trunk
Thoracic aorta
Superior mesenteric lymph nodes
Small intestine

hormones, and lipids. But when the lymphatic system has difficulty absorbing fats or transporting chyle, you may have some abdominal bloating. Or there may be more serious consequences, leading to chronic inflammation, weight gain, and other conditions described earlier.

The second function is to maintain a healthy environment in the digestive tract—which is critical in mounting a vigilant defense against food-borne infections. *Your gut lymphatics make up a whopping 70 percent of your immune system*, as you learned in chapter 1, and they produce white blood cells to defend your body against illness, making the gut/lymph node axis essential to the harmonious relationship between your intestinal microbiome and your immune system.

Though you likely know about the importance of what you eat to good gut health, chances are you haven't heard much about how the gut moves and flows, which is another reason lymph plays a pivotal role in digestive health.

The organs in your abdomen have a motility, or movement, essential to their proper function, called peristalsis. Peristalsis is the rhythmic, involuntary muscle contractions that move food through the digestive system, where nutrients are absorbed and waste is excreted. When organ motility is compromised—due to stress, inactivity, or nerve or hormonal dysregulation—digestive disorders can occur. The resulting symptoms include many of those my clients complain of when they come to see me: constipation, bloating, inflammation, and/or diarrhea. Abdominal self-massage can help alleviate these uncomfortable conditions because it encourages proper motility and helps absorb any leakage of blood capillary material from the small intestine. (You may have heard of leaky gut, a condition that can occur when there is inflammation of the villi in the small intestine, allowing food and toxins to escape into the bloodstream; this can trigger more inflammation and an unwanted immune response.)

If you have digestive issues, the "Abdominal Massage" sequence on page

122 can help relieve your symptoms. If you practice it regularly, you may even begin to find that you don't get sick as often, because you've cleared up congested lymph in the digestive tract. The "Deep Diaphragmatic Breathing" sequence on page 116 is also very therapeutic. It stimulates the contraction rate of your lymphatic system by approximately 15 percent, and this type of breath propels your lymph up toward your heart for recirculation into the bloodstream. I call this the *vacuum effect*. When I teach people how to massage their belly, I also encourage them to breathe deeply. This is a key reason people feel lighter and their pants feel looser after lymphatic drainage.

Your Other Digestive Organs

Your **liver**, located under your right rib cage, is an essential player in your lymphatic system. It breaks down fat and filters blood from the digestive tract before it goes to the rest of the body. This detoxifying and purifying organ also secretes bile, which is then transferred to the gallbladder, and manufactures proteins needed for blood plasma and other bodily functions. It detoxifies chemicals and drugs. It also produces an estimated 25 to 50 percent of the lymph that flows through your thoracic duct, which helps to regulate the immune system as well as retain proper fluid levels as it transports lymph back into your circulatory system. If your liver is unhealthy or diseased, there can be significant structural changes of the lymphatic vessels found within it. This compromises the lymphatic fluid levels and can actually increase your lymph volume—which is *not* what you want, as it can lead to lymphatic transport capacity overwhelm. With cirrhosis, for example, a common complication is that ascites can form. Ascites are an unusual accumulation of fluid in the cavity around the heart and lungs. If your lymphatic function isn't normal, interstitial fluid can build up, leading to lymphedema and ascites that can be overwhelming for your body to handle.

Your **gallbladder** is your liver's neighbor. It stores and concentrates the bile needed in the small intestine for digestion. Lymph from the gallbladder drains into the cystic lymph nodes, situated at the gallbladder's neck, which then empty to the hepatic nodes and finally to the celiac lymph nodes. When this pathway gets congested, bile salts (molecules secreted by the bile ducts that help digest fats) and bacteria can form gallstones.

Your **spleen** is your largest lymphoid organ. It's located under your diaphragm and left rib cage, near your stomach. It filters and stores your red blood cells and platelets in case your body needs them down the road, and your white blood cells, the keys to fighting infection. Your spleen and lymph nodes create invaluable lymphocytes (white blood cells) that produce antibodies to detect and kill dangerous bacteria, viruses, and pathogens to prevent the spread of an infection. Your spleen destroys old, defective red blood cells and is also responsible for maturing powerful antibody-producing B cells that have migrated there after forming in your bone marrow.

LYMPHATIC HEALTH = BRAIN HEALTH

Physiological Brain Health

Until very recently, little was known about the role of the lymphatic system in neurological health. In a fantastic discovery, the Danish scientist Maiken Nedergaard at the University of Rochester Medical Center identified the network of lymphatic vessels in the brain that eliminate toxins using cerebrospinal fluid. Nedergaard created the term **glymphatic system** (coining a word combining the brain's glial cells with "lymphatic" due to the system's dependence on glial cells). Her research was published in *Science Translational Medicine* in 2012. One of the most important results of her research was the discovery that the glymphatic system works primarily while we sleep (underscoring, yet again, the importance of uninterrupted sleep!).

Put simply, your glymphatic system functions as your brain's nightly bath. It uses the energy from the constant pulsing in your arteries to enable the exchange and drainage of waste products such as metabolites and proteins, and it connects to your brain's lymphatic system to flush this waste down and out of your body. Clearing out the gunk takes place twice as fast when you're sleeping as opposed 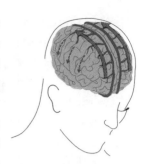 to when you're awake—which may be why we can't survive without regular sleep. These results support a new hypothesis to answer the age-old question of why sleep is necessary.

When the glymphatic system is inhibited, it has a harder time healing injuries and clearing out accumulated toxins in the brain, such as the amyloid plaque buildup that is a notable factor in dementia and Alzheimer's patients. Scientists at the Kipnis Lab at the University of Virginia Center for Brain Immunology and Glia are studying how aging impacts glymphatic vessel function. As we get older, the tiny lymphatic vessels in the brain narrow, making it harder for them to clear out waste. These researchers discovered that poor meningeal lymph drainage in the central nervous system can lead to cognitive impairments. They experimented with how to restore low-functioning lymphatic vessels in the brain, using a specific protein that acts as a growth factor to increase their diameter. When the diameter of subjects' lymphatic vessels was increased, they experienced better outcomes, including improved learning, memory, and glymphatic recirculation.

The evidence of this link between lymphatic health and brain health proves the vital role that lymph plays in a multitude of neurological diseases. Emerging science suggests that interventions incorporating the glymphatic system show promise in the treatment of Alzheimer's and Parkinson's diseases, other neuroinflammatory conditions, brain infections, and multiple sclerosis (MS). In fact, Antoine Louveau, a researcher at the Center for Brain Immunology and Glia (BIG) at the University of Virginia's Department of Neuroscience, recently observed, "Our data suggests that there is a signal coming from the brain to the lymph nodes that tells immune cells to get back into the brain, causing the [multiple sclerosis] pathology." Neurological conditions such as stroke, post-polio syndrome, and paralysis also show increased capillary pressure and fluid filtration, which can lead to swelling or lymphedema.

Hopefully, more research on these fluid dynamics in the brain will lead to novel therapies and treatments that could prevent or diminish the neurological and cognitive decline associated with aging. In the meantime, I recommend the headache sequence on page 99 and to get as much sleep as you can!

A Headache Story

One of my clients, Sergio, came to see me because he had been suffering from headaches, a common and painful symptom that he'd suffered from for many years, due in part, he believed, to having the MTHFR gene. MTHFR is the acronym for methylenetetrahydrofolate reductase, an enzyme that enables the body to process folate, or vitamin B_9. Methylation pathways govern detoxification and many important metabolic processes in the body, allowing the cardiovascular system, the neurological system, and brain chemistry to function properly. It also allows the body to detoxify toxins and heavy metals. If you have poor methylation, your body has a harder time processing the production of glutathione, the body's main antioxidant. When we become deficient in glutathione, we lose our natural defenses and are at a higher risk of developing autoimmune diseases, food sensitivities, and chemical sensitivities. Often people with the MTHFR gene get frequent headaches, have digestive issues, and have trouble losing weight.

In addition to having frequent headaches, Sergio was in an unhappy relationship and was having trouble sleeping—which you now know impacts the glymphatic system's ability to clear out waste in the brain. Once we started working together, he changed his diet and took supplements prescribed by a naturopath to support his methylation pathways and minimize his exposure to toxins. I saw Sergio each week, and he told me that his headaches were becoming farther apart. He also purchased an infrared biomat to help calm his nervous system to improve his sleep (more on biomats on page 300). Once his sleep improved, he gained enough confidence to speak up for himself in his relationship and things got better at home.

When Sergio recognized that lymphatic drainage massage was increasing his ability to detox, I showed him how to massage his head and neck and the corresponding lymph nodes. The entire sequence took no more than five minutes. I recommended he try it two or three times a week at first and see how he felt. A few months later, he told me that his headaches were gone and he had more energy and less mental fog. What had made the difference was that he had addressed his stress levels and developed a good nutrition plan in conjunction with lymphatic drainage. When people begin to work with their lymphatic system, they recognize that to maintain the benefits, they will be best served by cleaning up other areas of their life, too.

Emotional Brain Health

Lymph plays a role in how we feel mentally and physically every day. If we lack the ability to clean out waste in our brains, we suffer from brain fog, confusion, and a diminished attention span.

I encourage you to take a look at your internal and external landscape. In your physical body, this is about what you put into it (diet and nutrition), how much you exercise, and your past and current medical conditions. In your emotional body, this is about your relationships, family, work, past traumas, and burdens. Both the physical and emotional bodies are affected by the environment and even the changing of the seasons. All of these factors make up the full picture, or what I call the sociology of your health, and alter where you land on the lymphatic health continuum. Each element or input impacts the others.

One of my qigong teachers once told me that there's an entire universe in your abdomen. It contains the sun, the wind, the water, and all the elements necessary for optimal health. Our goal with self-massage is to create the intestinal equivalent of a perfect day—where the sun is shining, there's a slight breeze, and the humidity is comfortably low; just calm, clean, refreshing air. This environment will restore the motility and function of lymph flow in your internal organs and throughout your entire body, enabling your body to extract nutrients from your food and eliminate waste efficiently.

The beauty of lymphatic massage is that the more you support your lymph health, the more you clean out other areas of your life that cause stressors as well. It's similar to feng shui–ing your home, but for your body. Get your gut flowing by massaging your abdomen often, and you will probably feel much clearer, digest much better, and react to and deal with life's challenges much more easily. The self-massage sequences in chapter 4 will show you how to stimulate your abdominal organs to improve your metabolism so you can achieve a harmonious internal environment that will give you greater access to your energy.

THE TRADITIONAL CHINESE MEDICINE AND AYURVEDIC APPROACH TO HEALTH

One of the reasons I went into the healing arts was that I had studied the Chinese Five-Element Theory when I was in college. It was the first time I was introduced to the medical philosophy of tending to the body as you would a garden. To this day, I incorporate in my treatments the philosophy of *chi*—the flow of energy that runs through all living things. *Chi* flows through us and is considered vital energy that unites the body, mind, and spirit. When *chi* is flowing easily, we can enjoy good health. When *chi* is blocked or stagnant, problems can arise. The Chinese Five-Element Theory teaches that each of the organs of the body has a corresponding emotion.

Traditional Chinese Medicine and Chi Nei Tsang

In traditional Chinese medicine, each organ reflects an emotion. For instance, the liver is associated with anger, and one of its roles is "unclogging and deflation." The gallbladder, often referred to as "the general," is the decision maker of the body. If you're experiencing anger, irritability, impatience, rigidity, indecision, or nervousness, look to your liver and gallbladder underneath your right rib cage. The emotion attributed to the spleen is worry and

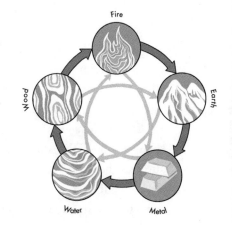

nervousness. If you find a situation challenging to digest or integrate, that can be an invitation for you to massage your abdomen under your left rib cage and acknowledge the need to nourish the message of your spleen.

When you begin to massage your abdomen, you may find a host of feelings trapped under your rib cage or pulling at your navel. My first lymphatic teacher placed a tremendous importance on working in the abdomen and incorporated techniques from chi nei tsang, a visceral massage method that applies the Taoist concept of qigong to release congestion in the vital organs; this improves digestion by stimulating lymphatic drainage and clearing emotional hurdles that impede organ motility. The techniques are so powerful that you will find them integrated into some of the steps in the "Abdominal Massage" sequence steps on page 122. Many of my clients have found trapped sadness or hidden workplace stress tucked into these crevices. Once these areas are tended to, you may feel a difference not only in your body but in your mind as well.

Ayurveda

When I was in high school in the 1980s, I started practicing yoga, which wasn't popular at the time. I found that it not only helped me emotionally, but I got stronger and more confident in my body. Later, while studying to become a yoga instructor, I learned about the five-thousand-year-old Indian system of holistic medicine called Ayurveda, meaning "the science of life."

One of the central Ayurvedic themes is understanding your *dosha*, or constitution. This is similar to the Chinese Five-Element Theory, which utilizes the various elements of nature to understand disharmony in the body. Ayurveda uses herbs, natural foods, exercises, and holistic modalities such as massage to help bring the body into balance. Even more fascinating is that Ayurveda has been talking about the lymphatic system

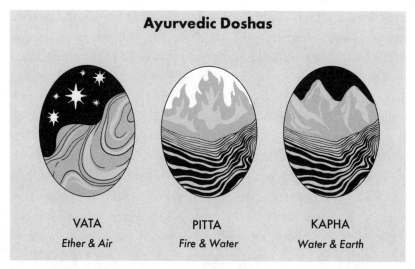

Ayurvedic Doshas

VATA
Ether & Air

PITTA
Fire & Water

KAPHA
Water & Earth

for centuries and recognizes the vital role it plays in health, especially in detoxification and preventing disease from taking root in the body. In many symptoms, Ayurveda looks to whether lymph is flowing freely; if not, it can be an indicator that the body isn't working efficiently. Rasa dhatu is the through line of primary waters of the body, including the interstitial fluid, lymph, blood, and plasma that your body depends on for optimal health; when the body's fluidity is restricted, it dries out and becomes more susceptible to developing illnesses, including digestion issues, skin issues, and mental fog. Doesn't that sound familiar?

Since Ayurveda uses specific herbs to promote healing and encourage lymphatic microcirculation in the body, you will find some of them listed along with more traditional Western herbs in chapter 5.

Chakras

I often look at how other cultures incorporate energy and emotions into treating the physical body. Energy can be explained in many ways. The chakras are energy centers of the body; translated from Sanskrit, the word means "wheel" or "disk." Also mentioned in ancient Hindu texts dating back to at least 1500 BC, the chakras are spiritual energy centers in the body that run from your spine to the crown of your head. Each chakra appears in a specific area and corresponds with specific organs and emotional or psychological states of being. Running through each chakra is *prana*, which means "life force" or "healing energy," which is similar to the concept of *chi* in traditional Chinese medicine. When you align with your chakras, you cultivate free-flowing energy through them, not unlike the flowing rivers of lymph that help clear the body.

I refer to the chakras in the self-massage sequences because you will notice that many areas of the body that you massage overlap with them. The ancient symbolism may be helpful for you to use during a guided visualization or to connect your emotional body with your physical body.

Although Western medicine often treats mental health as separate from physical health, practitioners in many other medical systems address the mind and body simultaneously to improve the well-being of their patients; this is referred to as a holistic approach to health. You may have experienced the way mental stress sets off your nervous system's fight-or-flight response and your body is immediately flooded with stress hormones. These hormones (cortisol and adrenaline, as well as thyroid and sex hormones) may help you manage the immediate threat, but if released consistently over time, they suppress your immune system— and a weakened immune system produces fewer lymphocytes to fight off potential infections. This is one of the reasons why you can feel so run-down physically and drained emotionally when you're stressed.

Meditation, visualization, and restorative yoga are effective ways to mitigate stress. In addition, the self-massage sequences in chapter 4 that target the brain have helped many of my clients achieve a calmer state of mind. I have found that these sequences boost energy, improve cognitive function, and help you feel more alert and focused. When you clear the stagnation in and around your head, you may feel as though an invisible veil has been lifted; this clarity will give you a greater ability to focus. My clients describe the feeling as being akin to turning on their windshield wipers: they suddenly feel clean and clear-headed. All of those positive feelings and symptoms are evidence that they have made beneficial changes deep inside their bodies, healing themselves from both outside in and inside out.

About Chakras

Each chakra has a corresponding emotion and color. You can connect with the chakras when you do self-massage by visualizing the color or meditating on the emotions associated with that region.

1st Chakra: Muladhara, Root Chakra
Located at the base of the spine and the pelvic floor
- **Emotions:** security, survival, feeling safe, foundation, financial security
- **Color:** Red

2nd Chakra: Swadhisthana, Sacral Chakra
Located just below your belly button
- **Emotions:** creativity, sensitivity, intimacy, sexual energy, self-expression
- **Color:** Orange

3rd Chakra: Manipura, Solar Plexus Chakra
Located between the navel and the sternum
- **Emotions:** self-worth, self-esteem, empowerment, confidence
- **Color:** Yellow

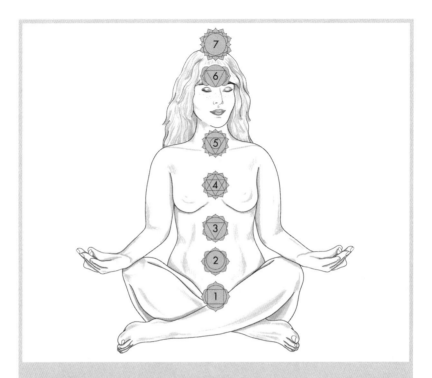

4th Chakra: Anahata, Heart Chakra

Located in the center of the chest

- **Emotions**: ability to give and receive love, compassion, empathy, self-love, healing
- **Color**: Green

5th Chakra: Visuddha, Throat Chakra

Located from the base of the throat to the center of the eyes

- **Emotions**: self-expression, communication, truth
- **Color**: Blue

6th Chakra: Ajna, Third Eye Chakra
Located at the center of the forehead between the eyebrows
- **Emotions:** wisdom, intuition, higher consciousness, imagination
- **Color:** Purple

7th Chakra: Sahasrara, Crown Chakra
Located above the head, like a crown
- **Emotions:** connects you to your higher self and highest purpose, purity, enlightenment, spiritual connection
- **Color:** Purple/violet

LYMPHATIC HEALTH = RESPIRATORY HEALTH

Adults take approximately fifteen to twenty breaths a minute. Babies inhale and exhale double that amount. Although breathing is automatic—a function of our parasympathetic nervous system—it's actually a complex process, and lymph plays a fascinating role in its function.

Your diaphragm, a thin muscle found underneath your lungs, is ceaselessly moving—just like your heart is constantly contracting as it pumps blood—to keep your lungs functioning. When you inhale, your lungs take in oxygen from the air. When you exhale, your lungs compress to remove carbon dioxide from the air you inhaled. This process is called gas exchange. If your breathing is too shallow, carbon dioxide accumulates inside your body; if this is very severe and chronic, it can lead to respiratory failure.

By taking a few deep breaths throughout the day, you are bringing oxygen to your lungs and improving your pulmonary respiratory system and your digestion. When you breathe deeply, the contractions in your

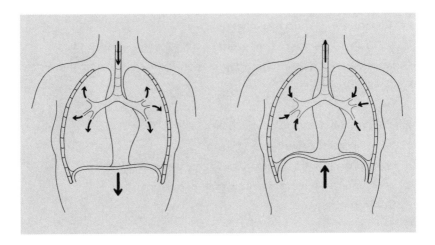

diaphragm alter the pressure in your chest that propels lymph from the lower half of your body up through the thoracic duct back to your heart. In addition, focusing on your breath is a form of meditation that has been shown to increase your parasympathetic rest-and-digest response, the state in which the body repairs itself and healing occurs.

Your lungs have a special way to protect themselves from toxins and bacteria. Cilia, which look like very small hairs, line your bronchial tubes. The cilia wave back and forth, spreading mucus into the throat so that it can be dispelled by the body. This cleans out the lungs and rids them of dust, germs, and any other unwanted items that may end up there.

The lymphatic system in the lungs monitors airborne particles and drains excess pathogen-containing fluid into the mediastinal lymph nodes found at your sternum. When you promote lymphatic drainage around your lungs, whether through deep breathing exercises or self-massage, you help your body remove excess toxins and drain accumulated fluid into your venous system for recirculation.

The lymphatic drainage pathways from your lungs are very complicated, moving through two interconnected sets of lymphatic ves-

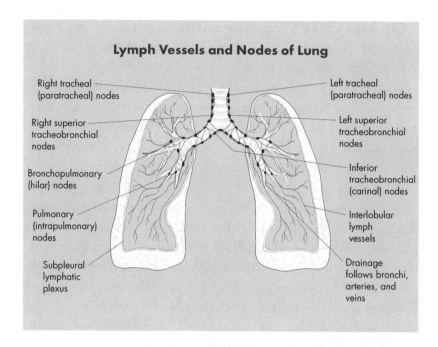

Lymph Vessels and Nodes of Lung

Right tracheal (paratracheal) nodes

Right superior tracheobronchial nodes

Bronchopulmonary (hilar) nodes

Pulmonary (intrapulmonary) nodes

Subpleural lymphatic plexus

Left tracheal (paratracheal) nodes

Left superior tracheobronchial nodes

Inferior tracheobronchial (carinal) nodes

Interlobular lymph vessels

Drainage follows bronchi, arteries, and veins

sels, called bronchomediastinal trunks. Lymph nodes inside the lungs and the mediastinum (the membranous partition between your lungs) do their filtering work, and then the lymph is returned into the blood through these vessels.

The essential function of lymph in the lungs is an intriguing topic for researchers. Recent studies have shown that changes to the lymphatic system are evident in nearly all lung diseases. According to the article "Lymphatics in Lung Disease," published by the National Institutes of Health in 2008, "The lymphatic circulation appears to be a vital component in lung biology in health and in disease. . . . Understanding the role of lymphatics in human lung disease appears likely to contribute to the understanding of the pathogenesis of disease and the development of novel therapeutic targets."

Ever since COVID-19 became a global pandemic in early 2020, people have been paying much more attention to their lung health. Infections in the lung are caused by viruses (which are hard to treat, as antiviral medications are often useless), bacteria (which often respond to antibiotics), fungal organisms, or toxins such as asbestos. A severe infection, such as the flu or COVID-19, can lead to pneumonia, which is an infection attacking the lungs' air sacs, or alveoli, which, when inflamed, become thick with mucus or fluid, making breathing difficult.

Some of the people hardest hit by COVID-19 are those with underlying health conditions such as diabetes, asthma, autoimmune disorders, chemical exposure, emphysema, pneumonia, and chronic obstructive pulmonary disease (COPD). Chronic smokers and breast cancer survivors who received radiation near their lungs are also considered to be more vulnerable. Those who survive COVID-19 can face a difficult recuperation, especially with their respiratory function and scarring in their lung tissue. As of this writing, scientists all over the world are looking into the blood lymphocyte levels of COVID-19 patients and how this new virus affects the production of lymphocytes in their immune response. Studies have shown low levels of blood lymphocytes, a condition called lymphopenia, in patients with severe COVID-19. A low lymphocyte count puts you at greater risk of infection and is typically associated with the development of cancer, AIDS, and repeated infections. Unraveling the role lymph plays in this virus may provide new insights for treatment.

Researchers are well on their way to investigating how the lymphatic system innately neutralizes pathogens by making antibodies. One researcher, Dr. Ziv Shulman at the Department of Immunology at the Weizmann Institute of Science in Rehovot, Israel, is an expert on how your body produces antibodies as part of the immune response to any infection. (Once you have antibodies, you are protected from developing the same disease again—the basis of how vaccines work.) According to an article on BioSpectrum, published in April 2020, "He and his lab were the first in the world to visualize all of the antibody-forming cells in intact lymph nodes. . . . This achievement, which shed new light on the 'how, what, when, and where' of the production of protective antibodies, revealed the lymph node niches—pockets in which antibodies undergo rigorous selection, so that only the most fit are sent off to target and bind to invading pathogens." The hope is that synthetic antibodies will be created—mimicking your body's lymphocytes—in order to be able to better fight off lethal pathogens, including COVID-19.

Until this happens or effective antiviral medications are developed, remind yourself daily of the invaluable role your lungs play in your health. My best advice is to tend to your immune health. Optimize the vitality of your lungs and your immune system so they remain strong. You can take simple steps to preserve cellular health and oxygen levels. A diet focused on anti-inflammatory foods (found in chapter 5) is an inexpensive way to change the composition of your lungs. Many herbs contain antioxidants and also have antibacterial and antiviral properties. I also encourage you to read about the benefits of eucalyptus in chapter 5; it's a great way to clear mucus in your lungs and open your air passageways. In addition, I developed the "Heart and Lung Opener" self-massage sequence on page 173, which will help the motility of your rib cage, based on the current knowledge of pulmonary lymphatics. There's also extensive information on how to breathe in the "Deep Diaphragmatic Breathing" sequence on page 116, which will increase oxygen flow in your body.

Using Lymphatic Self-Massage After Recovering from COVID-19

One of my virtual clients, Sunny, a woman in her fifties, reached out to me three months after recovering from COVID-19. Her overall health had stabilized, but she still had some lingering symptoms, including exhaustion and excess mucus in her chest. She had been cleared by her cardiologist of having any pulmonary issues but was looking for strategies to help support the health of her lymphatic system.

I explained how the lymphatic system clears congestion in the mucous membranes and the role it plays in respiratory health and told her that lymphatic massage had originally been developed to alleviate common colds and viruses. I recommended the "Heart and Lung Opener" sequence on page 173 as well as the "Sinus Congestion and Allergies" and "Abdominal Massage" sequences on pages 106 and 122. I also suggested a eucalyptus steam, regular Epsom salts baths, and anti-inflammatory herbs. Sunny wrote me two months later, telling me that she was doing the self-massage sequences three or four times a week and that my recommendations had been foundational in clearing out the stagnant remains of the virus. All of the practices I had recommended had become a mainstay in her health arsenal.

Now that you've gained a deeper understanding of the systemic nature of lymph flow—how it connects to all the systems and organs in your body and its essential role in facilitating immunity and the removal of excess inflammation—you're ready to learn the principles of self-massage. Remember that these sequences are rooted in science. When you work with your lymphatic system, you are working with your immune system, too. Because my education weaves together multiple cultural perspectives on healing the whole body, I invite you to incorporate specific, therapeutic imagery that you connect with into the self-massage sequences. When you take a multidisciplinary approach to health, you are promoting your physical, mental, and spiritual well-being from the inside out.

Part II

SELF-MASSAGE FOR INNER FLOW AND OUTER GLOW

Chapter 3

HOW TO BEGIN:
LYMPHATIC MASSAGE PRINCIPLES

Lymphatic self-massage utilizes the same massage techniques as a practitioner would but allows you to begin healing using your own two hands. This is a time to nurture yourself, to connect inwardly and set an intention to focus healing energy into your body. The sequences are based in science, but there is a mountain of research showing that anyone is capable of using touch for self-healing. Science shows that lymph flow increases during lymphatic massage. Thanks to fancy lymphangiography imaging called near-infrared fluorescence lymphatic imaging (NIRFLI) fueled by a green fluorescent dye (indocyanine green, or ICG) it's possible to map the increase of lymphatic uptake in real time during manual lymphatic drainage massage.

Touch is used to nurture people in nearly every culture; we just don't normally think to use it on ourselves. If you've ever rocked your child to sleep, held the hand of someone who was scared, or hugged a friend who was grieving, you know the power of touch. Lymphatic self-massage will connect your intuition to your innate biological process of healing *for yourself.* Remember, touch helps alleviate anxiety and stress and improves immune system function, sleep, pain, nausea, fatigue, and the side effects of chemotherapy. Touch can help wounds heal faster and alleviate symptoms of chronic conditions such as fibromyalgia, lupus, and many others.

Let those facts sink into your heart and mind before you begin. Allow yourself to be nourished! Your self-massage sessions are meditative acts of self-love and self-care. The more you practice this art, the more you will develop confidence, intuition, and a sensitivity to your body's needs like never before.

The self-massage strokes you'll be doing follow specific patterns toward lymph nodes to reduce inflammation. These sequences produce a *wavelike sensation* in your body, which creates the vacuum effect of absorbing fluid, flushing out toxins, and detoxifying your entire system. Your lymphatic network is so closely interconnected that when you work one area of your body, you can affect the lymphatic circulation in far-reaching parts of the system. The reason my method works so well is that you will be stimulating your lymph nodes—your lymphatic drains—before you do anything else.

I liken it to a dirty ring around your bathtub. If you're going to clean it, what's the first thing you do? Most people start scrubbing the ring. Others turn on the water. Actually, what you need to do *first* is clean the hair out of the drain. Otherwise, what's going to happen when you put water into the tub and scrub the dirty ring? It's going to back up with germ-laden fluid.

The same goes for your lymph nodes. By stimulating them *before* you push fluid toward them, they will be prepared to suction the fluid out of your tissues. This is why I encourage people to massage their lymph nodes prior to dry brushing. Remember, most of your lymph nodes are located in the hinges of your body. This seems designed to protect you and also for the nodes to receive as much movement as possible to function.

Let's take a look at the basics of how to do this.

PRINCIPLES OF SELF-MASSAGE

These guiding principles will enable you to enter deeply and safely into the sensory world of lymph as you learn lymphatic self-massage. Remember, your lymphatic fluid moves from your lymph nodes toward your heart. Keep the principles of the lymphotomes in mind as you do the sequences, and you will always be moving fluid in the right direction.

Tips for Starting a Sequence

1. **Massage your lymph nodes first.** Doing this is like sending out a signal to your body that you're about to flush toxins out of it. I joke with my clients that this is like the "Om" you say before beginning a yoga practice! *Lymph is everywhere*; it's systemic. When you first work your lymph nodes, such as those in your neck or armpits, you are preparing that area to receive lymphatic fluid. This is called "clearing the drains." Most sequences end with massaging the lymph nodes as well. Working the nodes as bookends solidifies the lymph's movement; you want it to peak in the middle and reinforce drainage patterns. This is why you'll repeat certain steps as you work your way back to the nodes you stimulated initially. Eventually you may even feel the effects in different areas of your body; for example, your arms and belly at the same time. You know you've hit the sweet spot when you hear a gurgle in your stomach, when the tenderness in a particular body part softens, or when you start to feel calmness wash over you.

2. **Massage gently!** Lymphatic self-massage should be *very* light. The

weight of the pressure should be a little more than
that of a feather but no more than that of a nickel or
dime. If you can feel your muscles, you're too deep.
If you've ever played air hockey, think about how the
puck moves across the table; lymph massage is just like
that. Let your strokes skim the surface just below your
skin; that's the magical plane where a lot of your lymphatic vessels collect excess fluid. At first it may feel
as though you're not doing much; that's *exactly* how it
should feel. (The exception is over the abdomen and
areas of cellulite, where you can use more pressure.)
If you've ever experienced the touch of cranial-sacral
therapy (a form of therapy that uses light touch to relieve compression in the head, spine, and sacrum from

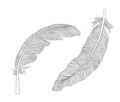
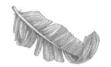

symptoms caused by the central nervous system), you know how light
your hands need to be. Going too deep won't harm you—but you
won't reap the benefits of a light touch.

3. **Cultivate a soft, nurturing touch.** Use the palms of your hands to *stretch
   the skin horizontally.* This is the secret of achieving a comforting,
   nourishing touch. You might be used to someone massaging you with
   knuckles or elbows during a more heavy-handed deep-tissue massage.
   That's the opposite of what you want to do here. Instead of pressing
   down, as most massage strokes do, try to work parallel to your skin to
   create a wavelike systemic motion. Imagine you're moving the foam
   of your cappuccino with your whole hand without pressing down into
   the coffee.

4. **Do not massage in a circular motion.** Your goal is to massage *one way*
   toward the lymph nodes. Have you ever seen how a caterpillar moves?
   It inches forward segment by segment. That's the technique you'll

be applying to ensure that you keep propelling lymphatic fluid properly. If you massage your-self in a circle, you are just putting fluid back to where you began. Instead, each stroke should be a half circle, or what I like to call a "crescent moon," or C-stroke, in honor of the shape. Your goal is to stretch your skin *lightly*—just a couple of inches—and then make a slight turn at the end of the stroke as if you're drawing the letter *C*. This is how to avoid making a full circle.

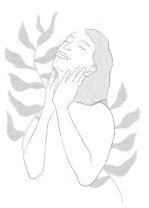

Contraindications to Self-Massage

Lymphatic massage of any sort is contraindicated if you have certain serious conditions. Consult with your physician before any sequences in this book if you suffer from active bleeding or blood clots, acute congestive heart failure, acute infection, acute renal failure, cellulitis, deep-vein thrombosis (DVT) or embolisms, or untreated cancer.

Precautions must also be taken and clearance from your physician obtained if you have any of these conditions: abdominal aortic aneurism, Alzheimer's disease and/or any other condition that requires the medical or psychiatric consent of an MD, an autoimmune disorder, bronchial asthma, cardiac edema or other heart conditions, diabetes, diverticulitis, hypersensitive carotid sinus, hypotension, multiple sclerosis, paralysis, phlebitic areas, pregnancy, presence of clot prevention devices, recent surgery and/or intra-abdominal scar formation following surgery, severe arteriosclerosis, thyroid dysfunction (Graves' disease, hyperthyroidism), vein inflammation, and/or pain with swelling.

5. **Work slowly.** Your lymphatic system moves at a snail's pace through your body. The vessel walls open and close to propel lymph about *six to twelve times per minute.* Your massage strokes need to be slow and light. Working with this rhythm is how you'll access the lymphatic fluid above the muscle 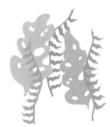 bed. It's what makes lymph massage extremely relaxing and effective, enabling your body to drop into the parasympathetic rest-and-digest mode. I often like to rock my body back and forth when I'm giving myself a massage, mimicking the ocean and creating a feeling of seaweed undulating in the waves.

6. **Know which direction to go in.** Check the Lymphotomes map first (see p. 7)! Be sure which lymph nodes drain the area you plan to massage. Understand which territories of your body correspond to which set of lymph nodes before you start a sequence.

7. **Use skin-to-skin contact as much as possible.** Place your hands directly on your skin. You can stimulate the lymph nodes over your clothes, but when you touch your bare skin, you get to know your internal landscape, your body's peaks and valleys, and sticky spots on it. You'll feel the consistency of your fluid change as you work. Your skin contains nerve endings that will provide valuable feedback. You don't need to use oil; you will get a better stretch of your skin without it. (The exceptions are the "Improve Cellulite" and "Athletic Injuries, Pre- and Postoperative Recovery, and Scar Tissue" sequences on pages 140 and 232.)

8. **Get comfortable.** For most sequences, whether you are sitting, lying down, or standing up, make sure you are comfy. I specify which position to be in only if it's essential to that particular sequence. I recommend massaging directly on your skin, but the best kind of clothing to wear is something loose and comfortable with a breath-

able fabric. Be sure to ditch the underwire or sports bras when you're working on yourself.

9. **Breathe deeply.** When you breathe deeply, you create deeper contractions of your diaphragm. This acts as an external pressure on the largest lymph vessel—your thoracic duct—which brings lymphatic fluid from the lower half of your body and limbs up toward your heart. It's as simple as expanding your belly when you inhale and relaxing your belly when you exhale.

10. **Hydrate!** Our bodies are approximately 70 percent water; basically, we're aquariums! Increasing the amount of water you drink will help circulate immune cells, nourish your lymph vasculature, and flush out toxins. Proper hydration also helps your skin glow. Aim for at least nine eight-ounce glasses of water each day, more when it's hot outside. Herbal tea is included in that count.

    Another way to calculate how much you should hydrate is by multiplying your weight by two thirds (thats 67%) to one ounce of water for each pound you weigh. So if you weigh 150 pounds, you should drink about 100 ounces of water. Always drink clean, filtered water. I recommend starting your day by drinking a glass of warm water with a squeeze of lemon in it. Keep drinking plenty of water throughout the day, especially if you're practicing lymphatic self-massage. Water will help move out debris from your tissues.

11. **Note your progress.** As you continue your self-massage practice, I encourage you to try new sequences and keep a journal to note how you feel afterward. You may find a shift in your emotions and your perspective. Remember what I said in the Introduction: *Energetically, lymph represents the flow of life.* When you clear your internal engine, you may notice your mood changing. I often practice a sequence if I'm in a bad mood or feeling melancholy; it's one of the fastest ways I know to improve my physical and mental health simultaneously.

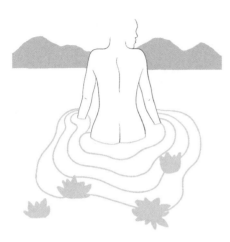

Whenever possible, set aside a quiet time in which to integrate the work after your sequence. Some people feel light and bright afterward, while others feel tired and wiped out. Moving toxins through the body isn't always comfortable at first. Lymph will continue to circulate for a while after you're done. It's not uncommon to feel the effects well into the next couple of days. You are accessing your ability to heal, and your immune system will respond.

How Lymphatic Massage Reduces Swelling

Several years ago, I was called to work on a woman in her seventies who had been diagnosed with amyotrophic lateral sclerosis (ALS, also known as Lou Gehrig's disease). Her disease had progressed to the point that she was confined to a wheelchair and needed round-the-clock care. Since she wasn't walking anymore, her feet had become very swollen and purple. Her wife, a physician, thought lymphatic drainage might help reduce her swelling. When I first met with her, I decided that it would be best to keep her in her wheelchair and teach her wife and caregiver how to administer lymphatic massage sequences themselves.

I began by teaching them the science of how lymph flows. I massaged each regional lymph node group, what I refer to as "clearing the drains," to systemically stimulate her entire lymphatic system. I first massaged the right and left lymph nodes at her neck—the main drains. Next, I massaged the **axillary lymph nodes** under her armpits. Then I did the breathing sequence in her abdomen. Finally, I worked on the **inguinal lymph nodes** at the top of her thighs that the fluid from her feet and legs drain into—and guess what happened? The color in her feet returned to normal! The purple color vanished before our very eyes! **By working the lymph nodes first, you create a suction effect so lymphatic fluid can drain easily.** I hadn't even touched her lower legs or her feet yet, but her feet were now the same flesh tone as the rest of her body. Fortunately, her wife had been recording the session on her phone, because we were all truly amazed.

When you stimulate your lymph nodes before you work on the area of fluid you want to move, you will engage your entire system.

BASIC STROKES FOR LYMPHATIC SELF-MASSAGE

The specific strokes of lymphatic self-massage are designed to mimic the waves of automotoricity, the physiological pulse that propels lymph. Your goal is to stretch your skin in a nurturing manner. There are several types of strokes for lymphatic self-massage.

With all your strokes, you want to have a working pressure and a resting pressure to avoid massaging yourself in a circle.

The **working pressure** is the active movement of your stroke—your grip and stretch of the skin.

When you release your grip, the skin rebounds on its own. This is the **resting pressure**.

The exception is when you're working on your abdomen.

The C-Stroke

With this stroke, you simply want to stretch your skin *lightly*—just a couple of inches—and then make a slight turn at the end of the stroke, drawing a *C* or crescent moon on your skin. By massaging yourself this way, you ensure that lymphatic fluid moves toward your drains instead of creating the 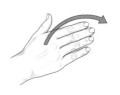 backflow that would occur if you massaged your skin in circles. Another way to think of the crescent moon is that you're making a long *C* motion. Remember to finish your stroke by aiming the fluid toward the lymph nodes.

The J-Stroke

Similar to the C-stroke, the J-stroke is a long stroke with a small tail at the end that curves off at the end, like the letter *J*. The J-stroke starts off many of the head and neck sequences with the steps that massage the right and left supraclavicular lymph nodes above the collarbone.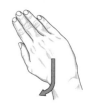

Overlapping C-Strokes

This stroke is mainly for your abdomen, when it's okay to make full circles with your hands over your colon and navel.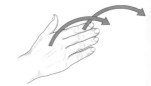

The Rainbow Stroke

The rainbow stroke is an upside-down C-stroke. You will use this stroke over your breasts, chest, arms, and legs. The same principles apply, and I'd like you to imagine that you are infusing yourself with the hope and optimism of a rainbow.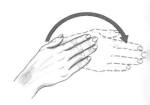

The Pump Stroke

The pump stroke uses the palm of your hand between your index finger and your thumb. Most of
the power of this stroke comes from your palm and
the heel of your palm. This stroke is helpful on limbs
and large areas of the body, such as your arms, armpits, legs, and thighs. It's a wonderful way to broadly
move a large swath of fluid.

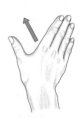

Think of the way seaweed undulates in the ocean. When the waves
are calm, the seaweed can expand effortlessly and move with freedom.
When the waves speed up, the seaweed gets tangled and remains stationary and stagnant. Always move slowly, with intention.

The "Spock" Sequence

The "Spock" sequence is so powerful and used in
many sequences that it deserves some extra attention. If you've ever seen *Star Trek*, you know that
the character Spock's famous salute, "Live long and
prosper," is accompanied by a hand gesture in which

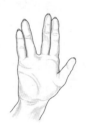

he separates his fingers between his middle and ring fingers. That finger
separation is the basis of this stroke. Place your middle finger, index
finger, and thumb behind your ear and your ring and pinky fingers in
front of your ear. (If it's more comfortable, you can separate your fingers
between your index and middle fingers.) *Gently* massage in front of and
then behind your ear at the same time. Aim the fluid simultaneously
toward the back of your head and down your neck toward the lymphatic
nodes at the base of your neck. This will help release the fluid that builds
up around the ears. This stroke is very powerful to do before and after
you have a cold and for ear congestion, a hangover, sinus pressure, and
more.

Swallowing During Sequences

Saliva doesn't just moisten your food to help you swallow; it also kills bacteria in your mouth and begins the digestive process. When you swallow, the food and saliva enter the esophagus, where smooth muscle movements (called peristalsis, which you learned about in chapter 2) move them toward the stomach.

Saliva is formed in the salivary glands inside your cheek and around your jaw, mouth, and teeth (the parotid, submandibular, and sublingual glands). In fact, new scientific research points to another set of salivary glands located in the nook where the nasal cavity meets the throat; the glands connect the ears to the throat—the muscles involved when you swallow. You will be encouraged to swallow when you do massage strokes around your ear to stimulate the smooth muscle contractions associated with draining fluid in your sinuses from your head and neck through your lymphatic system.

The Shirt-Collar Lymphatic Zone

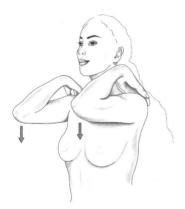

This is the lymphatic zone where your shirt collar is located—the area at the top of your shoulders. The lymphatic drainage pattern goes from the back of your neck and wraps around toward the front of your neck, where it empties into the right and left supraclavicular lymph nodes above your collarbone. To stimulate your shirt-collar lymphatic zone, place both hands on top of your shoulders at the trapezius, your elbows pointing straight in front of you. Inhale, then exhale and drop your elbows, keeping your fingertips on your shoulders.

Chapter 4

LYMPHATIC SELF-MASSAGE SEQUENCES

Now that you've become acquainted with the lymphatic system and its incredible impact on your health and well-being, you're ready to learn how you can optimize the function of your lymph using your own two hands with a series of simple massage techniques targeted to address specific imbalances. The sequences in this chapter are designed to enable you to be your own nurturer and healer.

At the beginning and end of each sequence you will stimulate your lymph nodes. You will be instructed to repeat the same steps to create a suction effect, similar to the way you would clear a drain. Certain strokes also reappear in multiple sequences because the drainage patterns of lymph are similar across regions of the body. This is the secret of the routines: work your lymph nodes first, then move fluid into them. It's that simple.

Keep in mind that most of your lymph nodes reside in the hinges of your body. Nodes are clustered under your armpits, in your neck and abdomen, and in the creases of your thighs not only to safeguard them but also to benefit from your movements throughout the day, whether you're walking, turning your neck to look around, or reaching for things dozens of times per day. They are your foundational drains. You will use at least one set of them in each sequence. All of the small movements in the sequences help propel lymph. Once you are familiar with the lymphatic map, your intuition can take over.

After a couple tries, these routines will sink in and you'll feel as though you've been doing them your whole life. Each step takes only a few seconds and each sequence just a few minutes. I like to refer to images from nature—rainbows, waterfalls, crescent moons, oceans of seaweed, and rays of sun—so you can plant those calming images in your mind as you give yourself the gift of self-care.

Remember, your body is saturated in lymph; you have about twice as much of it as you do of blood. As you practice these self-massage techniques, try to feel the rivers of lymph bathe your cells and tissues in bacteria-fighting goodness. Imagine you are submersing yourself in a protective white sheath of health. I also encourage you to enhance the benefits of your new routine by drinking plenty of water, making healthy food choices, and regularly doing exercise you love. These habits will allow your lymph to keep flowing, flush out toxins, and boost your immune function.

At the end of each sequence, you'll see a series of icons that correspond to the holistic remedies and exercises in chapter 5. Adding those supportive elements into your self-care routine will help you achieve an ideal balance of eliminating impurities and avoiding overburdening your lymphatic system. Taking a multimodal approach is the best way to achieve lymphatic health and enjoy its many regenerative benefits.

NOTE: Unless specifically stated, all sequences should be done in whatever position is most comfortable for you: sitting, standing, reclining, or lying on a yoga mat or bed.

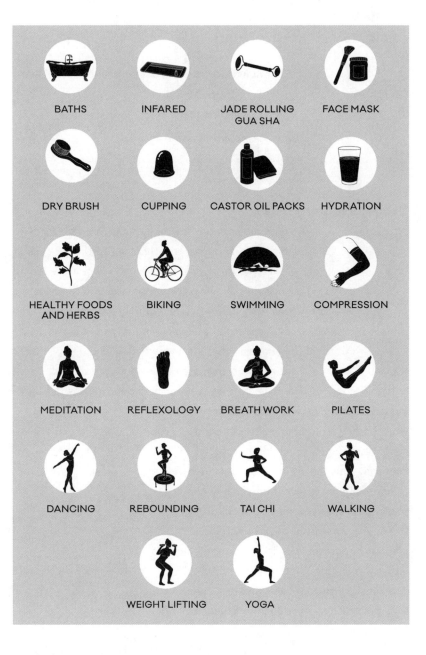

BATHS

INFARED

JADE ROLLING
GUA SHA

FACE MASK

DRY BRUSH

CUPPING

CASTOR OIL PACKS

HYDRATION

HEALTHY FOODS
AND HERBS

BIKING

SWIMMING

COMPRESSION

MEDITATION

REFLEXOLOGY

BREATH WORK

PILATES

DANCING

REBOUNDING

TAI CHI

WALKING

WEIGHT LIFTING

YOGA

COLD-LIKE SYMPTOMS

Congestion/Sore Throat

Earache

Headache

Sinus Congestion and Allergies

Congestion/Sore Throat

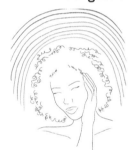

Have you ever noticed how vulnerable your throat is to illness, particularly during the changing of the seasons or right before you get a cold? Maybe you've felt the lymph nodes in your neck swell. The lymph nodes in the neck are often palpable when you're fighting an infection—and when this happens, it's usually the first time people realize that they have a lymphatic system.

There are approximately one to two hundred lymph nodes in your head and neck; they're your first defense against fighting the bacteria and viruses that enter your body through your mouth and nose. Your mouth, for example, is full of bacteria. Your tonsils are large clusters of lymphatic cells (also known as lymphoid organs, as you learned in chapter 1). They're located in the pharynx and play an important role in your immunity by ensuring that foreign matter doesn't slip into your lungs and respiratory system. They produce antibodies

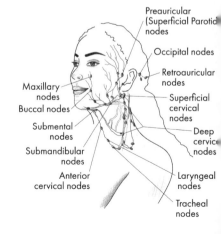

to combat viruses and then flush them out via the lymph. There is lymph in the roots of your teeth and on the surface tissue of the base of your tongue, too.

Using Ayurveda for Congestion/Sore Throats

*In Ayurveda, there's a concept called **ama**. It refers to unmetabolized waste, an accumulation of toxins that can clog and weaken the channels in the body. It's said that when ama is not regularly cleared and elimi-nated, it becomes the cause of disease. Although different doshas man-ifest the disharmony with varying symptoms, an accumulation of ama in the digestive tract or respiratory system makes you susceptible to colds, phlegm, and mucus in the lungs and sinuses. Fluid buildup can affect your ears, nose, throat, lungs, and bowel movements. If you get a cold and are feeling sluggish and run-down, pay particular attention to your diet; you'll see a list of foods to eat on pages 272–75, a list of anti-inflammatory herbs on page 279, and a list of foods to avoid on page 276 (especially dairy products, meat, and gluten).*

I use this sequence on myself all the time and have been teaching it to my clients for years. It's most effective right when you feel a cold coming on, as a canker or herpes cold sore develops, or when you're starting to cough and sneeze and your throat is sore. I developed this protocol to keep you healthy and enhance your body's natural cleansing and protective functions.

One of my clients is a woman in her late eighties with a social life more active than mine; she is constantly at risk of catching a cold or flu due to her exposure to other people. But she rarely gets sick. She always tells me it's because she's diligent about strengthening her immunity with lym-phatic self-care.

Evidence shows that stress is a contributing factor to illness. We all get sick from time to time, so when that happens, look into what is depleting you. If you notice the lymph nodes in your neck swelling, think about the strains you are under and where you can minimize the pressure you're feeling. When you have too much going on, it's easy to feel overwhelmed and think you can't carve out time to take care of yourself. Make sure you get enough sleep! It's one of the simplest and most affordable ways to benefit your immune system.

When you start to feel that little tickle in your throat or if you've been eating too much sugar, drinking too much alcohol, or otherwise overindulging in less-healthy foods and beverages, use this sequence to clear out debris and stimulate the antibacterial enzymes in your saliva to keep the ecosystem of your mouth in balance. I practice this sequence two or three times a day when I'm feeling run-down; that feeling is an early indicator that my body needs support. The more you practice self-massage, the more in tune you'll be with your body and able to sense when it needs a boost. It's so effective that I hope you will incorporate this sequence into your routine when the weather begins to shift or after you've had the flu to clear out mucus and congestion.

NOTE: Do not do this sequence if you have an acute infection or swollen lymph nodes as a result of infection. Wait until the infection is cleared before you massage yourself, and consult your physician before doing so. If you have swollen lymph nodes in your neck that don't go away, consult your physician. Some lymph nodes remain swollen for long periods of time due to past dental infections, underlying chronic conditions (such as herpes), or trauma to the area. Have the area imaged if your doctor deems it necessary.

Step 1

Stimulate the right and left supraclavicular lymphatic nodes at the base of your neck just above your collarbone. Press your fingertips **down** into the hollows above your collarbone. Make a **J** motion as you press **lightly down** and **out** toward your shoulders. Repeat ten times.

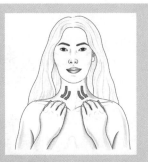

Step 2

Perform the "Neck" sequence. There are three steps:

1. Place both your palms at the base of your neck. Pulse the skin **gently** as you stroke **downward** toward your collarbone. Repeat ten times.
2. Place your hands higher so your pinky fingers rest in the groove behind your ears, your fingertips pointing diagonally toward your ears. Use your palms to stretch the skin **downward** toward your neck. Repeat five times.
3. Make light brushstrokes from behind your ears all the way down your neck. Repeat five times. Swallow once.

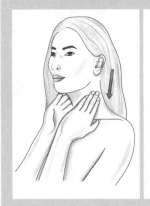
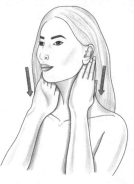
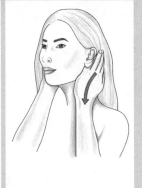

Step 3

Perform the "Spock" sequence: Separate your fingers between your middle and ring fingers (Spock-like). Place your middle and index fingers behind your ears in the cartilage groove and your ring and pinky fingers in front of your ears. **Gently** massage **back** and **downward** in a C-stroke. Repeat ten times. This stimulates both the pre- and retroauricular lymph nodes of your ears. This should be a rhythmic, nurturing movement. Swallow once.

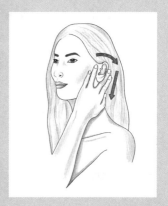

Step 4

Place your hands behind your ears, your pinky fingers resting in the cartilage groove. **Gently** glide the heels of your hands **downward** in a C-stroke. Repeat ten times.

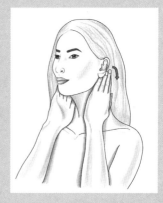

Step 5

Stimulate your shirt-collar lymphatic zone: Place your hands on top of your shoulders, your elbows pointing straight in front of you. Inhale, then drop your elbows as you exhale, keeping your fingertips on your shoulders. Repeat five times. This helps move lymphatic fluid from the back of your neck to the drains above your collarbone.

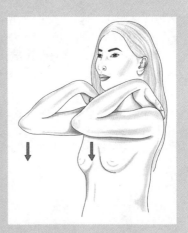

Step 6

Repeat Step 3, the "Spock" sequence. Swallow once.

Step 7

Place your fingertips at the base of your skull, in the occipital ridge. With your fingers touching, **gently** walk your fingertips along this ridge, then glide them **down** your neck, the way a waterfall streams down a mountain. Repeat ten times.

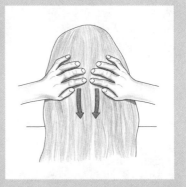

Step 8

Repeat Step 5: Stimulate your shirt-collar lymphatic zone.

Step 9

With the pads of your fingers, massage overlapping C-strokes from your chin to your earlobes. This is the drainage pattern for the teeth (submental nodes), salivary glands, mouth, lips, and tongue (submandibular nodes). This area also contains the reflexology zones for your colon and stomach, which often gets congested when you have a cold. Repeat three times.

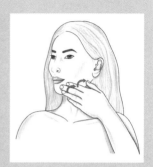

Step 10

With the pads of your fingers, massage C-strokes horizontally from the top of your cheeks to your ears. This will stimulate your parotid nodes (which drain your nasal cavity) and tonsillar lymph nodes (which drain your tonsils). It's also the reflex area for your colon and heart, which can benefit if there's any ama accumulation here. Repeat five times.

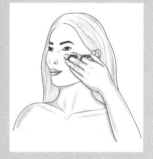

Step 11

Place the pads of your middle fingers on either side of your nostrils. Hold **lightly** for a few seconds; then, using all your fingertips, sweep along underneath your cheekbone to your ears. This is the reflex area for your lungs. Repeat five times.

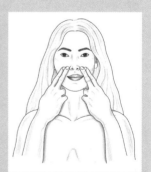

Step 12

Make light brushstrokes along your face from your cheeks to your ears and from the top of your nose to your forehead and out to your ears. Repeat three times.

Step 13

Massage from the bridge of your nose straight up your forehead to your hairline five times. This is the reflex area for the liver and gallbladder.

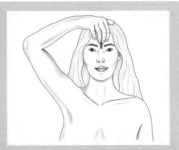

Step 14

Run your fingers along your hairline to your temples five times. Then massage C-strokes at your temples. Repeat five times.

Step 15

Open your mouth wide. Take a deep breath in. Exhale with a strong "Whoooo." This is the sound associated with the stomach and spleen. Repeat three times.

Step 16

Repeat Step 3, the "Spock" sequence, to clear the congestion in and around your ears. Swallow once.

Step 17

Drop your right ear to your right shoulder. Hold for three seconds, breathing in and out. Drop your left ear to your left shoulder. Hold for three seconds, breathing in and out. Repeat twice. If you are comfortable, make small circles with your head, rolling it around your shoulders. Reverse the direction. Breathe. Swallow twice. Stretching your neck will clear tension and stagnation in the neck that may be interfering with lymph flow.

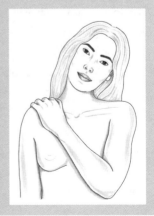

Step 18
Repeat Step 2, the "Neck" sequence.

Step 19
Repeat Step 7: Massage the occipital ridge at the base of your skull.

Step 20
Repeat Step 5: Stimulate your shirt-collar lymphatic zone.

Step 21
Repeat Step 1: Stimulate the right and left supraclavicular lymphatic nodes at the base of your neck.

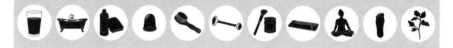

Earache

If you're prone to earaches or allergies or to developing waxy or fluid buildup in your ears, this sequence is for you. If you've recently gotten over a cold, this sequence will move out the extra fluid that is clogged inside the ears. In the summer when I swim a lot, this is my go-to sequence to clear out any fluid residue.

My clients love this sequence for the clarity it brings to their hearing. It also helps clear up sinus issues and alleviates symptoms of temporomandibular joint dysfunction (TMJ), a tightness in the jaw that can cause pain and difficulty eating. It's subtle but powerful. Hearing loss experts will tell you that stress plays a role in diminished hearing because it disrupts the blood circulation. You may also know that your ears are the location of your body's motor control (vestibular) system, which maintains your balance and posture and allows you to walk without falling. The fluid canals in your inner ear are involved in moving your muscles and joints and even in feeling the sensations in your hands and feet.

The lymph drainage patterns of the ear ultimately go to the supraclavicular right and left lymphatic nodes at your collarbone. Lymph from your ears drains into the preauricular and retroauricular nodes in front of and behind your ears—which is why I love the "Spock" stroke so much. It's important to stimulate the occipital ridge at the base of your skull and behind your neck to encourage lymph flow down the back of your neck.

Finally, when you look at the emotional aspect of this work, think about the noise of the outside world compared to your inner voice. How can you be more compassionate with yourself? I invite you to listen to your inner self as you do this sequence. Tuning in to your inner voice may help you feel more clear-headed.

If you wear earrings, avoid pulling on them. You may want to remove them before performing this sequence. I've found in my practice that some people develop metal allergies as they age. Take notice if this is something you may be experiencing.

NOTE: If you experience multiple or chronic earaches, consult your physician or an ear, nose, and throat specialist.

How to Resolve an Earache and TMJ at the Same Time

A virtual client named Zion reached out to me because he recently had an ear infection. Although the acute infection had cleared, he kept experiencing earaches throughout the day that started in the morning after he woke up. He also told me that he had been living with jaw pain for years due to TMJ from grinding his teeth during sleep, despite wearing a night guard. On top of that, he had recently had some painful dental work done and was swollen and having difficulties opening his jaw. I showed him the pathways of lymph drainage around and behind the ear and down the neck (which are located at the hinges that open and close the jaw). I taught him how to do the "Earache" sequence, and we stayed in touch via email. After a couple months of consistent self-massage practice, he told me that he was beyond amazed: not only had the chronic earache gone away, but his jaw felt better because the lymph massage had helped release muscular tension that was hindering lymph flow. Many people are taught to massage the jaw muscles deeply when there's TMJ, but that can trigger the opposite response and create more inflammation. When you take a mild approach to the musculature in the face, you can create a more harmonious environment for the muscles to soften while keeping the lymph flowing. After doing this self-massage sequence, Zion was able to fully open his jaw again and his pain was significantly reduced. He texted me, "My mind is blown by this!"

Step 1

Stimulate the right and left supraclavicular lymphatic nodes at the base of your neck just above your collarbone. Press your fingertips **down** into the hollows above your collarbone. Make a J motion as you press **lightly down** and **out** toward your shoulders. Repeat ten times.

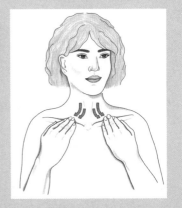

Step 2

Perform the "Neck" sequence. There are three steps.

1. Place both your palms at the base of your neck. Pulse the skin **gently** as you stroke **downward** toward your collarbone. Repeat ten times.
2. Place your hands higher so your pinky fingers rest in the groove behind your ears, your fingertips pointing diagonally toward your ears. Use your palms to stretch the skin **downward** toward your neck. Repeat five times.
3. Make light brushstrokes from behind your ears all the way down your neck. Repeat five times. Swallow once.

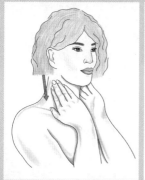
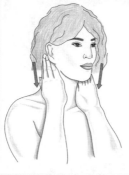
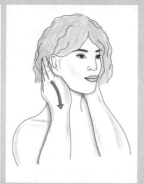

Step 3

Perform the "Spock" sequence: Separate your fingers between your middle and ring fingers (Spock-like). Place your middle and index fingers behind your ears in the cartilage groove and your ring and pinky fingers in front of your ears. **Gently** massage **back** and **downward** in a C-stroke. Repeat ten times. This stimulates both the pre- and retroauricular lymph nodes of your ears. This should be a rhythmic, nurturing movement. Swallow once.

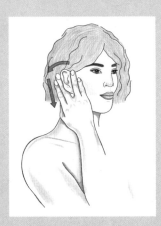

Step 4

Place your hands behind your ears, your pinky fingers resting in the cartilage groove. **Gently** glide the heels of your hands **downward** in a C-stroke. Repeat ten times.

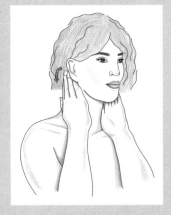

Step 5

Place your fingertips at the base of your skull, in the occipital ridge. With your fingers touching, **gently** walk your fingertips along this ridge, then glide them **down** your neck, the way a waterfall streams down a mountain. Repeat ten times.

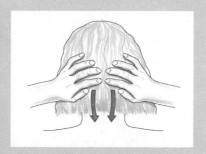

Step 6

Repeat Step 3, the "Spock" sequence. Swallow once.

Step 7

Make light brushstrokes from behind your ears down your neck. Repeat three times.

Step 8

Stimulate your shirt-collar lymphatic zone: Place your hands on top of your shoulders, your elbows pointing straight in front of you. Inhale, then drop your elbows as you exhale, keeping your fingertips on your shoulders. Repeat five times. This helps move lymphatic fluid from the back of your neck to the drains above your collarbone.

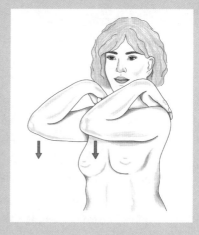

Step 9

Shoulder stretch: Place one hand on the opposite shoulder, resting your forearm diagonally across your chest. Drop your elbow as you stretch your neck toward your ear, breathing deeply. Repeat five times. Repeat on the other side five times.

Step 10

Repeat Step 3, the "Spock" sequence. Swallow once.

Step 11

Do ear pulls:

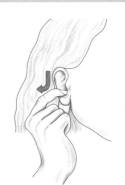

1. With your index finger and thumb, *gently* stretch the cartilage inside your earlobe **downward** and **outward**, toward the back of your head. Hold for ten seconds, breathing deeply. Release your ear, open and close your mouth twice, and swallow once.
2. Move your index finger and thumb to another spot inside your earlobe. *Gently* stretch the lobe **downward** and **outward**, toward the back of your head. Hold for ten seconds, breathing deeply. Release your earlobe, open and close your mouth twice, and swallow once.

3. Continue working all along your earlobe up to the very top of your ear. *Gently* stretch the cartilage in each place **outward** toward the back of your scalp, and hold for ten seconds. (If you are wearing earrings, be mindful to avoid them.)

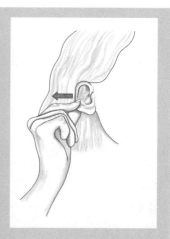

4. Make tiny C-strokes inside the very top of your ear, where the cartilage is thin. Continue stroking **downward** and **outward**, directing the fluid away from your face.

5. With your index finger inside your ear, grab the small pointed nodule in front of your ear where it meets your cheek, called the tragus. Pull in toward your cheek. Hold for ten seconds. Move the nodule up and down and back toward your cheek again. Release your ear, open and close your mouth twice, and swallow once.

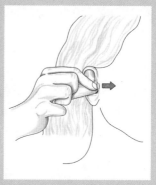

6. Place your fingers on your upper cheekbone in front of your ear. Make tiny C-strokes up toward your hairline, over your ear, and then down your neck. Repeat five times.

Step 12
Repeat Step 11 on your opposite ear.

Step 13

Make light brushstrokes along your face from your chin to your ears, from your cheeks to your ears, and from your forehead to your ears. Repeat three times.

Step 14

Repeat Step 3, the "Spock" sequence.

Step 15

Repeat Step 5: Massage the occipital ridge at the base of your skull.

Step 16

Make light brushstrokes down the back of your neck toward your collarbone. Repeat five times.

Step 17

Repeat Step 9: Stretch your neck: Tilt your ear down toward your shoulder. Breathe deeply in and out as you hold the stretch for ten seconds before you release. Repeat on the opposite side of your neck. Do twice on each side. Make circles with your neck if it's comfortable.

Step 18

Repeat Step 2, the "Neck" sequence.

Step 19

Repeat Step 1: Stimulate the right and left supraclavicular lymphatic nodes at the base of your neck.

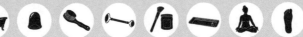

Headache

I developed this sequence after I learned about the groundbreaking discovery of the glymphatic system in the brain discussed in chapter 2. Recent studies have shown that the lymphatic vessels surrounding the brain
play an important role in neuroinflammatory diseases and brain infections.
The glymphatic system, which gets its name from the glial cells and the
lymphatic system that it mimics, explains how the lymphatic system works
with cerebral spinal fluid to clear excess fluids, solutes, and waste products from the brain via lymphatic vessels when we sleep.

Neuroscientists have discovered that the lymphatic vessels in the brain
help clean out amyloid plaque (the clumps of protein that occur in abnormal amounts in Alzheimer's patients and that are responsible for the
disruption of cell function), which makes the case for a good night's sleep
even more urgent. Over time, these lymphatic vessels narrow, making it
more difficult for them to clean the debris from the neurons so they can
function and communicate effectively.

I cannot emphasize the importance of this discovery enough. Directors
at the NIH believe that cures for neurological disorders may come from
studying the link between the glymphatic system and the cleaning out of
cell debris in the brain. Good lymphatic health is essential to good brain
health!

As researchers develop ways to treat narrowing lymph passageways,
you can do your part with self-massage, given the principles you know
about how lymphatic vessels respond to touch and movement. You will notice your headaches, dizziness, and brain fog improve with this sequence
because you are increasing the absorption and transportation rate of cellular waste. I've had wonderful outcomes with this protocol with clients
who suffer from migraines, stress headaches, diseases such as Lyme disease, and autoimmune conditions such as lupus that trigger headaches.

Before you begin, remember that the right side of your head drains to the right supraclavicular lymphatic nodes, and the left side of your head drains to the nodes on the left. As you move through this sequence, picture the fluid clearing out debris similar to the way water sweeps out the leaves in rain gutters, creating a pathway for fresh water to flow effortlessly.

Step 1
Stimulate the right and left supraclavicular lymphatic nodes at the base of your neck just above your collarbone. Press your fingertips **down** into the hollows above your collarbone. Make a **J** motion as you press **lightly down** and **out** toward your shoulders. Repeat ten times.

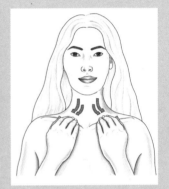

Step 2
Perform the "Neck" sequence. There are three steps:

1. Place both your palms at the base of your neck. Pulse the skin **gently** as you stroke **downward** toward your collarbone. Repeat ten times.

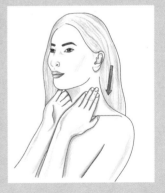

2. Place your hands higher so your pinky fingers rest in the groove behind your ears, your fingertips pointing diagonally toward your ears. Use your palms to stretch the skin **downward** toward your neck. Repeat five times.

3. Make light brushstrokes from behind your ears all the way down your neck. Repeat five times. Swallow once.

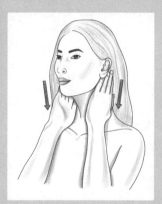 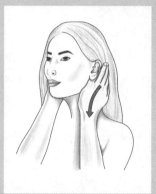

Step 3

Perform the "Spock" sequence: Separate your fingers between your middle and ring fingers (Spock-like). Place your middle and index fingers behind your ears in the cartilage groove and your ring and pinky fingers in front of your ears. **Gently** massage **back** and **downward** in a C-stroke. Repeat ten times. This stimulates both the pre- and retroauricular lymph nodes of your ears. This should be a rhythmic, nurturing movement. Swallow once.

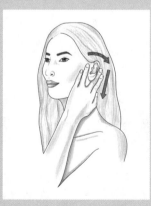

Step 4

Stretch your neck: Draw your ear down toward your shoulder. Breathe deeply in and out as you hold the stretch for ten seconds before you release. Repeat on the opposite side of your neck. Repeat twice on each side. Make circles with your neck if it's comfortable.

Step 5

Inhale, squeezing both shoulders up to your ears. Exhale, releasing your shoulders. Repeat five times.

Step 6

Place your fingertips at the base of your skull, in the occipital ridge. With your fingers touching, **gently** walk your fingertips along the ridge, then glide them **down** your neck, the way a waterfall streams down a mountain. Repeat ten times.

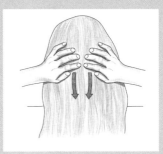

Step 7

Stimulate your shirt-collar lymphatic zone: Place your hands on top of your shoulders, your elbows pointing straight in front of you. Inhale, then drop your elbows as you exhale, keeping your fingertips on your shoulders. Repeat five times. This helps move lymphatic fluid from the back of your neck to the drains above your collarbone.

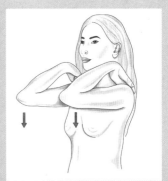

Step 8

Lightly brush your face with your fingers from the chin to the ears. Make long brushstrokes from your cheeks to your ears and from your forehead to your ears. Repeat three times.

Step 9

Massage your scalp with your fingertips as if you're shampooing your hair. Massage your entire head toward the back of your scalp and down the back of your neck to stimulate the glymphatic system in your brain. Visualize your brain as a clean, bright light.

Step 10

Draw rainbows on your scalp. There are three steps:

1. Place your right hand on top of your head at the center of your scalp. Make "rainbows" with the heel of your hands down the right side of your scalp to move the fluid toward the back of your neck. Stop just behind your right ear. Repeat five times. Repeat on the left side five times.
2. Place your right hand a little farther down on your scalp and closer to your ear. Make "rainbows" with the heel of your hand **downward** toward the back of your neck. Repeat five times. Repeat on the left side five times.
3. Place both hands on the top of your head, closer to the occiput at the base of your skull. With the heels of your hands, make C-strokes all the way down the back of your neck. Repeat five times.

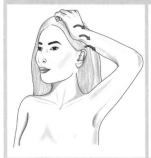
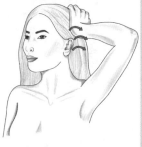
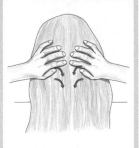

Step 11

Place your hands behind your ears, your pinky fingers resting in the cartilage groove. **Gently** glide the heels of your hands **downward** in a C-stroke. Repeat ten times.

Step 12

Repeat Step 3, the "Spock" sequence.

Step 13

Massage small C-strokes at your temples, the spot people rub when they have a headache. You can find it by opening your mouth and closing it so that your teeth touch; the muscle on the side of your forehead will move. This is a wonderful area to massage if you grind your teeth and have TMJ, but please be gentle and loving here! Repeat ten times. Swallow once.

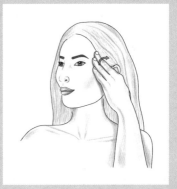

Step 14

Repeat Step 10: Draw rainbows on your scalp.

Step 15

Repeat Step 9: Massage your scalp with your fingertips as if you're shampooing your hair.

Step 16

Repeat Step 6: Massage the occipital ridge at the base of your skull. Swallow twice.

Step 17

Repeat Step 8: Make light brushstrokes along your hairline, forehead, and face.

Step 18

Repeat Step 4: Stretch your neck.

Step 19

Circle your head slowly in each direction. If you are prone to vertigo, skip this step.

Step 20

Do shoulder lifts: Lift your shoulders toward your ears. Inhale, hold your breath for three seconds, then exhale and relax your shoulders. Repeat five times.

Step 21

Rub your palms together vigorously. Once they heat up, place them over your eyes. Hold them there for ten seconds as you breathe deeply. As you release your hands, press your palms into your cheekbones.

Step 22

Repeat Step 7: Stimulate your shirt-collar lymphatic zone.

Step 23

Repeat Step 1: Stimulate the right and left supraclavicular lymphatic nodes at the base of your neck three times.

     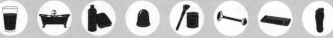

Sinus Congestion and Allergies

Sinus congestion and allergies are very common. Your sinuses are cavities in your skull and the bones of your face are covered with a thin layer of mucus, part of the respiratory tract that extends from your nose to your throat. They are air-filled sacs, empty spaces that filter and clean the air that flows into your nose up through your sinuses and down into your lungs. Whether you have struggled with sinus issues for years or developed symptoms later in life, your sinuses are connected to your brain, so it's essential to keep the passageways clear from infection.

Sinuses are found in your face and even in the back of your head. **Maxillary sinuses** are found on both sides of your nostrils near your cheekbones. Above your eyes near your forehead, including the eyebrows, are your **frontal sinuses**. On each side of the bridge of your nose near your eyes are your **ethmoid sinuses**. Behind the ethmoids are what's called the **sphenoid sinuses**, which is why you will be massaging along the line at the base of your skull (the occipital ridge).

Your sinuses need to be able to drain freely. Allergies, infections (which produce extra mucus), and other irritations can inflame the sinus tissue and narrow the air passageways, causing pain. Inflammation can affect the frontal sinuses around your eyes and the bridge of your nose, which explains why you may sometimes get sinus headaches.

If your sinus issues are a result of allergies, you may benefit from allergy testing to pinpoint the source of your allergic response. The culprit may be airborne, for example pollen, or it might be something in your diet or environment. Sinus symptoms may also be the result of a deviated septum in your nose, which inhibits breathing.

Whatever the cause of your sinus problems, this sequence is designed to open the sinus cavity, drain excess mucus, and clear the lymphatic path of drainage down your neck. I encourage you to swallow during some of the sequences to stimulate the smooth muscle contractions that occur when you drain fluid in the head and neck.

When you massage certain points in your head, you can relieve pressure and pain you may have around your cheekbones, jaw, and neck. Some of my clients notice that their sinus issues arise from situations other than environmental exposure that they can't quite explain. I often ask them if they recently had dental work done, because bacteria in your mouth can make its way to your sinuses. I also encourage them to take an inventory of their emotional landscape. Your thoughts are formed in the prefrontal cortex of your brain, which is just above your sinus cavity. Often, mental stress creates muscular tension that puts a strain on this area—which may resonate with you if you find that, energetically speaking, your thoughts are stifling your imagination.

Step 1

Stimulate the right and left supraclavic-ular lymphatic nodes at the base of your neck just above your collarbone. Press your fingertips **down** into the hollows above your collarbone. Make a **J** motion as you press **lightly down** and **out** toward your shoulders. Repeat ten times.

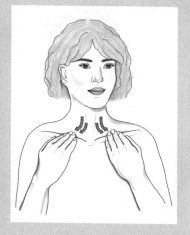

Step 2

Perform the "Neck" sequence. There are three steps:

1. Place both your palms at the base of your neck. Pulse the skin **gently** as you stroke **downward** toward your collarbone. Repeat ten times.
2. Place your hands higher so your pinky fingers rest in the groove behind your ears, your fingertips pointing diagonally toward your ears. Use your palms to stretch the skin **downward** toward your neck. Repeat five times.
3. Make light brushstrokes from behind your ears all the way down your neck. Repeat five times. Swallow once.

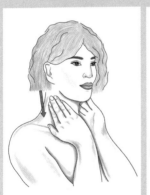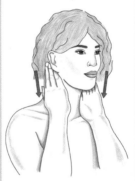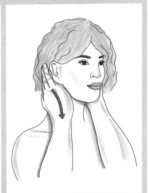

Step 3

Perform the "Spock" sequence: Separate your fingers between your middle and ring fingers (Spock-like). Place your middle and index fingers behind your ears in the cartilage groove and your ring and pinky fingers in front of your ears. **Gently** massage **back** and **downward** in a C-stroke. Repeat ten times. This stimulates both the pre- and retroauricular lymph nodes of your ear. Swallow once.

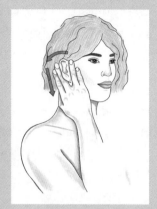

Step 4

Place your fingertips at the base of your skull, in the occipital ridge. With your fingers touching, **gently** walk your fingertips along this ridge, then glide them **down** your neck, the way a waterfall streams down a mountain. Repeat ten times.

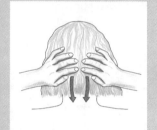

Step 5

Stimulate your shirt-collar lymphatic zone: Place your hands on top of your shoulders, your elbows pointing straight in front of you. Inhale, then drop your elbows as you exhale, keeping your fingertips on your shoulders. Repeat five times. This helps move lymphatic fluid from the back of your neck to the drains above your collarbone.

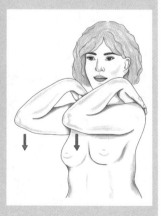

Step 6
Lightly brush your face with your fingers from the chin to the ears, from your cheeks to your ears, and from the bridge of your nose up to your forehead and out to your ears. Repeat three times.

Step 7
With the pads of your fingers, massage overlapping C-strokes from your chin to your earlobes. This is the drainage pattern for the teeth (submental nodes), salivary gland, mouth, lips, and tongue (submandibular nodes). Repeat three times.

Step 8
With the pads of your fingers, massage C-strokes from your cheeks to your ears. This will stimulate your parotid nodes (which drain your nasal cavity) and tonsillar lymph nodes (which drain your tonsils). Repeat three times.

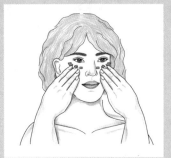

Step 9
Place two fingertips beside each nostril where your sinuses are located. Press lightly down and out. This will drain the fluid in your nasal cavity. Please be very gentle when touching the fluid just underneath your skin. Resist the urge to press too deeply. Breathe deeply, inhaling through your nose and exhaling through your nose (if you're not too congested). Repeat five times.

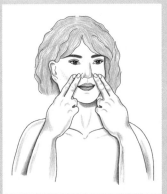

Step 10

Place your fingers a little higher up on the side of your nose. Press **lightly down** and **out**, holding the stretch of the skin for ten seconds and breathing deeply. Repeat three times.

Step 11

With the pads of your fingers, **gently** tap from your nose to your cheekbones to your ears. Repeat five times.

Step 12

Make light brushstrokes from the base of your nose and cheeks to your ears.

Step 13

Place your fingertips under your eyes, fanning your fingers out. **Lightly** press into your skin and hold for three seconds, breathing deeply. You will feel the very top of your cheekbones here. Press **very gently** along the top line of your cheekbones to your ears. Repeat five times.

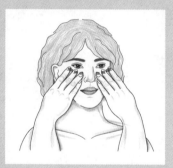

Step 14

Tap your fingertips on the tops of your cheekbones toward your temples. Repeat five times.

Step 15

With the pads of your fingers, massage C-strokes **lightly** along your temporal bone where the tops of your cheekbones and your ears meet. Repeat five times. Swallow once.

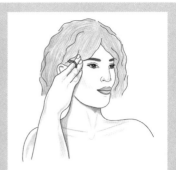

Step 16

Massage up the center of your eyebrows into your forehead, where your third eye and sixth chakra, the center of intuition, are. This is a great point for your sinuses and allergies (and the Botox line!). Repeat five times.

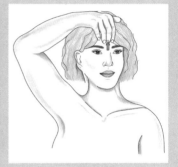

Step 17

Place your middle fingers at the inner end of each eyebrow. **Gently** pinch and lift your eyebrows. Hold for ten seconds. Repeat twice.

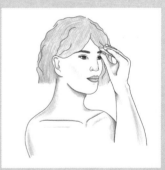

Step 18

Pinch and lift two more spots on your eyebrows: the middle and the outer end. Repeat twice.

Step 19

Make gentle brushstrokes along your eyebrows to move fluid toward the tops of your ears. Repeat three times.

Step 20

Massage each side of your forehead toward your ears. Massage the very top of your forehead at your hairline. Repeat five times.

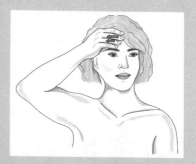

Step 21

Repeat Step 15: Massage your temples **gently** with C-strokes. Repeat ten times.

Step 22

Repeat Step 6: **Lightly** brush your face with your fingers from the chin to the ears, from your cheeks to your ears, and from the bridge of your nose up to your forehead and out to your ears. Repeat three times.

Step 23

Repeat Step 4: Massage the occipital ridge at the base of your skull. Then make light brushstrokes behind your ears and down your neck.

Step 24

Repeat Step 3, the "Spock" sequence.

Step 25

Repeat Step 2, the "Neck" sequence.

Step 26

Repeat Step 1: Stimulate the right and left supraclavicular lymphatic nodes at the base of your neck.

NOTE: I recommend a facial steam, nasal irrigation, or warm washcloth compress afterward.

DIGESTIVE HEALTH

Deep Diaphragmatic Breathing

Abdominal Massage

Digestive Issues

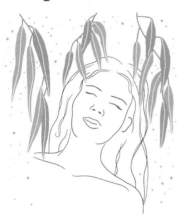

From the food we eat to the stress we're under to the medications we take, our gastrointestinal health often falls victim to the realities of modern living. But maintaining a balanced gut is essential to good immune health as well as optimal digestion and a glowing complexion.

Bloating and digestive issues are a top concern for a majority of my clients. It's probably the box that is checked the most often on my new-client intake form. As discussed in chapter 2, gut inflammation is prevalent today. This is in no small part a result of our consuming poor-quality food, chemicals, and antibiotics, though stress also takes a toll on our bellies. My clients routinely say, "Most of my food is organic, but I'm still bloated all the time." Nearly all of them admit to being chronically stressed, which is often the hidden cause of their digestive issues.

Western culture sees massaging the abdomen as taboo, which is a shame since most of our vital organs and several lymphoid organs are located in the belly. It's the source from which we all sprang; we literally developed outward from our umbilical cord at our navel. Our small intestine, colon, liver, spleen, stomach, and gallbladder all have intrinsic movement and motility, called peristalsis, necessary for optimal functioning. These organs can become impacted and made sluggish by stress, food, and lifestyle. Many people suffer from constipation or irregularity and worry.

When I went to college, my digestion became very sensitive due to hormonal changes, stress, and unhealthy dorm cafeteria food. No matter what I ate, I got bloated. If I dared to look at chocolate, it seemed as though I gained five pounds. One of the reasons I became a lymphatic practitioner was the relief I got from lymphatic drainage treatments in massage school. Not only did they reduce the bloating in my gut, my acne cleared up, too. After lymphatic treatments, I immediately felt lighter, with more energy and vitality.

Throughout my career, I've helped many clients deal with chronic inflammation by using lymphatic drainage techniques in the abdomen. Because the liver, gallbladder, spleen, colon, and small intestine all play a role in elimination, it's crucial that you develop an understanding of your anatomy to harmonize lymphatic flow in this area. The self-massage techniques in this sequence are designed to alleviate tension that adheres to your gut, promote the healthy functioning of the digestive tract, increase fat absorption, reduce inflammation, and calm stress and anxiety.

How to Get Rid of Belly Bloat

Maxine, in her midthirties, came to see me on the recommendation of an integrative physician she'd been seeing because she believed her work stress was the cause of her constipation and bloating. She admitted that she wouldn't be able to change her job anytime soon, and she knew she had to address her digestive issues. She admitted that she holds a lot of stress and emotions in her belly. She told me she used to get constipated in high school before exams. She also experienced stomachaches in large social gatherings and in the workplace.

Although Maxine had struggled with constipation for decades, even after she changed her diet, she started to wonder if there was a connection between her stress levels and her digestion because she noticed that her stomach didn't bother her when she was on vacation or when she wasn't feeling overwhelmed with responsibilities. After each of our sessions she texted me with a happy poop emoji, exclaiming with joy when her bowels moved. I taught Maxine how to do diaphragmatic breathing and how to massage her belly so she could do it on her own in between appointments. I also made sure she was drinking plenty of water throughout the day so she wasn't dehydrating her lymphatic pathways. A few months later, she told me that her constipation was gone and she had even lost a few pounds! Her bloating had also dissipated, and she often used the breathing techniques I had taught her. With those tools, she told me, she felt better equipped to deal with the stress she faced at work.

Deep Diaphragmatic Breathing

Most of my clients aren't breathing. Of course they are breathing, but they're not really b r e a t h i n g. Shallow chest breathing—what most of us are used to doing—isn't the same as diaphragmatic breathing. As you read earlier in the book, deep diaphragmatic breathing is one of the most effective things you can do to help move your river of lymph from the lower half of your body and legs up the thoracic duct toward your heart. Your **lumbar lymph nodes** are located between your diaphragm and pelvis. Those nodes drain the pelvic organs and abdominal wall. Try visualizing the lymph vessels in your GI tract cleansing, absorbing fat, and eliminating waste as you practice the deep breathing technique. To stimulate the motility of your digestive system, follow these simple steps. This sequence will help you feel calmer and more peaceful in a matter of minutes.

Step 1

Lie down in a comfortable position. Place your hands on your abdomen. Make sure your elbows are relaxed. If you have the space, prop pillows under your arms so there's absolutely no tension in your body. Relax your jaw, throat, and forehead.

Step 2

Take a long, deep breath, expanding your belly into your hands as though you're blowing up a balloon. Count to five as you inhale. As you exhale, count backward from five and let your stomach relax. Inhale again. As you exhale, feel the back of your body soften into the surface beneath you. Repeat five times.

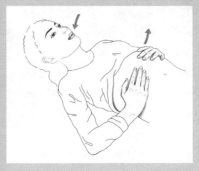

Step 3

Breathe into the sides of your torso. Feel your breaths fill both sides of your rib cage with air. Exhale and feel your ribs soften. Repeat five times.

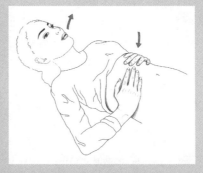

Step 4

Inhale higher now, bringing the breath all the way into your chest. Allow your breath to lift your front from your stomach to your sternum. Feel the expansion into your heart and breastbone. Imagine the colors of the third and fourth chakras, yellow and green, filling your chest. Exhale slowly and think about letting go of whatever no longer serves you. Repeat five times.

Step 5

Inhale all the way up to your shoulders, filling your heart and your lungs with air. Exhale slowly, allowing the back of your body to softly relax into the surface beneath you. Repeat five times.

Step 6

The M-breath and spiral technique: You're going to breathe into nine places in your abdomen. You will do two full inhales and exhales for each hand position. As you exhale, spiral your fingers down into your belly. You'll be using a firm pressure—deeper than in previous massage strokes—and the action will be vertical, not horizontal. 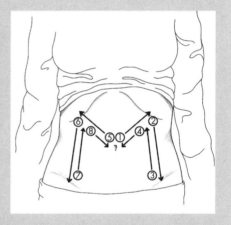 The nine hand positions will form an M shape on your belly, which will help release the *ama* in your colon.

1. The first hand position is directly over your navel. Take a big breath in, and expand your breath into your navel. As you exhale, make spiraling circles with your fingers straight down into your belly. Follow your breath downward. Repeat once.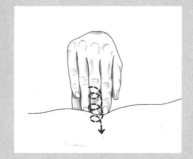

2. Second hand position: Move your hand under your left rib cage (stomach and spleen location). Inhale to this spot. As you exhale, circle your fingers deeply down into this spot. Repeat once.

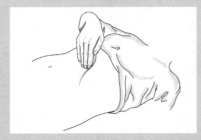
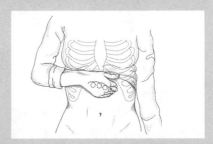

3. The third hand position is in front of your left hip (descending colon location). Push your breath up into your hand as much as possible, then exhale and circle your fingers down into the soft spot in front of your hip. As you grow more accustomed to breathing this way, you can provide

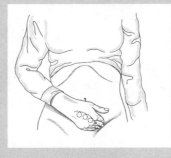

resistance with your hands on the inhale and corkscrew your hands deeper toward your spine on the exhale. Repeat once.

4. The fourth hand position is under your left rib cage again. Repeat Step 2: Resist your breath on the inhale, and, as you exhale, make spiraling circles down into your abdomen under your left rib cage. Repeat once.

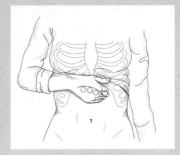

5. The fifth hand position is over your navel again. Repeat Step 1: Breathe with resistance into your navel; as you exhale, spiral your fingers downward into your stomach. Repeat once.

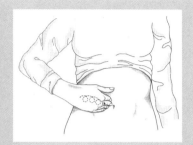

6. The sixth hand position is under your right rib cage (liver and gallbladder location). Inhale here and resist your breath with your hand. As you exhale, make circles with your fingers down into your abdomen just below your right ribs. Repeat once.

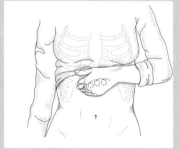

7. The seventh hand position is in front of your right hip (ascending colon location). Push your breath up into your hand as much as possible, then exhale, circling your fingers down into the soft spot in front of your hip. Provide resistance with your hand on the inhale, and corkscrew your hand deeper toward your spine on the exhale. Repeat once. You will feel your inhales growing larger now. You may feel tenderness on your exhales as you spiral your fingertips into your abdomen.

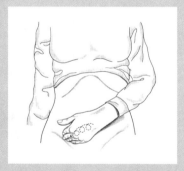

8. The eighth hand position is at your right rib cage again. Repeat Step 6: Resist your breath on the inhale, and, as you exhale, make spiraling circles down into your abdomen under your right rib cage. Repeat once.

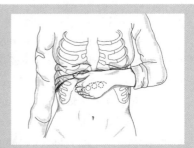

9. The last hand position is at the navel again. Repeat Step 1: Expand your breath into your navel. As you exhale, make spiraling circles with your fingers down into your belly. Follow your breath downward. Repeat once.

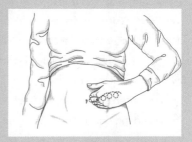

Step 7
Take a few cleansing, normal breaths. Relax the skin of your forehead. Feel your eyes recede into their sockets. Allow your bones to sink heavily into the surface beneath you. **Smile.**

It can be hard to move your breath all the way up your body at first. Don't be discouraged. The more you take the time to tend to this area, the more you will feel the gentle wind of your breath greet you.

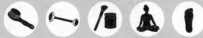

Abdominal Massage

I created this sequence to benefit your digestion. The more you practice this technique, the more it will alleviate bloating and the inflammatory process so you can have that "five pounds lighter" feeling.

Bloating can be caused by many factors, including a less-than-optimal diet, stress, hormones, illness, menstrual cycle, medications, vitamin deficiency, food allergies, lack of sleep, and an imbalance in the gut microbiome. Diet pills and diuretics aren't helpful because your lymphatic system requires hydration to circulate. Diuretics are dehydrating, which can lead to stagnant, congested tissues and sluggish lymph.

Who touches your belly? Hardly anyone. Maybe your mother when you were a child, maybe your lover. That's it. When your stomach hurts or if you've eaten too much, you instinctively clutch your belly for relief. I believe this is an indication that you need touch! With lymphatic self-massage, you can harmonize your digestive tract by encouraging the peristalsis in your gut so it has the movement necessary to absorb nutrients, secrete (the

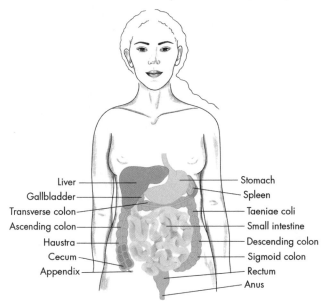

Liver — Stomach
Gallbladder — Spleen
Transverse colon — Taeniae coli
Ascending colon — Small intestine
Haustra — Descending colon
Cecum — Sigmoid colon
Appendix — Rectum
— Anus

organs of the pancreas, liver, and gallbladder secrete hormones such as insulin, enzymes, and bile to aid in digestion), and function optimally. As you read in chapter 2, the lymphatics in your gut make up 70 percent of your immune system, so caring for your gut also promotes good immune health.

Stress and tension can get lodged in the belly. The Chinese Five-Element Theory states that each organ has a corresponding emotion: liver (anger), gallbladder (irritability, indecisiveness), stomach and spleen (worry), lungs (sadness, grief), heart (joy), and kidneys (fear and creativity). Looking at health from a mind/body/spirit point of view is now a part of most holistic health practices. When you integrate your emotions into your healing, you can see the toll that negative emotions take on your body.

I've studied visceral massage techniques from various cultures and incorporated those concepts into this sequence to help you balance your emotions and address your physical discomfort. This sequence will help you alleviate constipation, minimize your bloating and acid reflux, and strengthen your immunity. Just like a back rub, a few simple lymphatic massage strokes can melt the tension in your viscera and stimulate an ideal environment for eliminating waste.

One of the most valuable gifts you can give yourself is nurturing self-love and acceptance. Rubbing your belly is a part of self-care.

Step 1

Stimulate the right and left supraclavicular lymphatic nodes at the base of your neck just above your collarbone. Press your fingertips **down** into the hollows above your collarbone. Make a **J** motion as you press **lightly down** and **out** toward your shoulders. Repeat ten times.

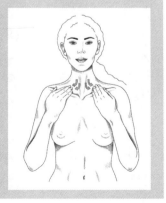

Step 2

Stimulate the inguinal lymph nodes: Place your hands on top of your inner thighs. Massage C-strokes **upward** to the crease at the top of your thighs. Repeat ten times. Repeat on your outer thighs.

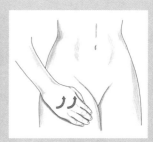

Step 3

Lie down so you're comfortable. You can place a pillow underneath your knees to soften your abdomen and release your back muscles. Place your hands flat on your stomach. Breathe deeply three times. As you inhale, feel your stomach rise. As you exhale, feel your belly fall. Visualize the anatomy of your digestion. Your colon is shaped like an upside-down **C**. You're going to massage your abdomen with your whole hand in circles following the lines of elimination. Your ascending colon runs from your right hip up to your right rib cage. Your transverse colon crosses above your na-

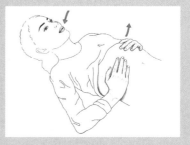

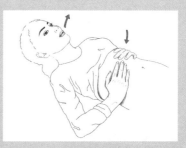

vel from the right rib cage to the left rib cage. Your descending colon goes from your left rib cage down toward your left hip. Then your colon makes a slight turn under your belly button before descending to your rectum.

Step 4

With the palms of your hands, make overlapping circles all around your colon: up the right side, across your abdomen, and down your left side. Use a little more pressure here, about the amount you would use when rolling out dough to make pizza. Make circles under your navel toward your left hip to continue the motion. Imagine you are drawing suns and moons all over your abdomen. Visualize a clear sky in your

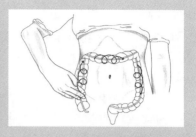

belly, radiant with moonlight and sunshine. Allow your strokes to be nourishing and simple. Use as much of your palm and fingers as possible. Knead your skin like a pawing cat. Feel the terrain. Notice where your hands are drawn to go and where they are keen to avoid. Release judgment or the urge to work aggressively toward an outcome. Shift your focus to self-love and acceptance, softening the landscape. Bring comfort to the area with loving, gentle, compassionate hands. Invite acceptance and awareness. Allow this to be an invitation to opening. Feel the surrounding tissue start to melt underneath your hands. Circle your abdomen at least ten times.

Step 5

Massage small overlapping circles around the circumference of your belly button. Make sure you massage around your abdomen at least ten times, but you can do more if you feel like it. You can use a little more pressure here, as

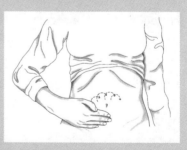

this is where your deeper lymphatic network resides. If you find any tight areas, spend some quality time nourishing yourself here.

Step 6

Make light brushstrokes from the four corners of your abdomen to the center of your abdomen ten times from each corner to your navel.

Step 7

Repeat Step 4: Massage your colon five times.

Step 8

Using the outer edge of your hand, scoop your abdomen in front of your hip bones toward your navel. Begin in front of your right hip bone. This is where your cecum, ilium, ileocecal appendix, and the beginning of your ascending colon are located. It's also the area where your small intestine 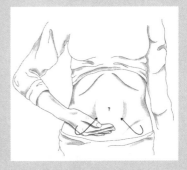 merges into your large intestine (colon). This can be tender or tight if you've had long-standing chronic constipation. Use your palm to scoop from the front of your right hip toward your navel. Next, scoop in front of your left hip bone toward your navel. This is the end of your descending colon, where your sigmoid colon meets your rectum. This side can be tender if you've recently been constipated, so be gentle here. You don't want to stretch the skin—that can be painful! You can create slack in your skin by pushing toward your hip first, then massaging **down** into your belly, then toward your navel. Repeat five times on each side.

Step 9

Using the outer edge of your hand, scoop underneath both sides of your rib cage toward your navel. Your liver and gallbladder are located under your right rib cage, close to where your ascending colon bends to become your transverse colon. **Gently**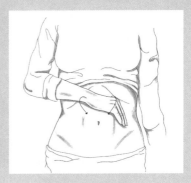

create slack in the skin first, then scoop **downward** and **outward** from your rib cage toward your navel, similarly to Step 8. Your stomach and spleen are located under your left rib cage. This is near the splenic flexure or bend from the transverse colon to the descending colon. Contour your palm underneath your rib cage and pump **downward** and **outward** toward your navel. Repeat five times on each side.

Step 10
Repeat Step 4: Massage your colon three times.

Step 11
Do navel pulls around your belly button. This is wonderful to help alleviate small tensions and misalignments in the abdomen from patterns that put strain on the muscles and organs. With the fingertips of one hand, **gently** pull

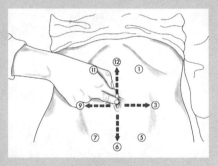

the edges of your navel **outward**. Use whichever fingertips are most comfortable for you. To begin, pull straight **upward** as though your navel is a clock and the time is 12:00 (this point corresponds to the heart). Stretch and hold the skin for at least one minute in each spot while you breathe in and out. Then move to 3:00 (the left kidney), 6:00 (the bladder and genital organs), 9:00 (the right kidney), and any other "time" that needs your attention; for instance, 1:00 (stomach and spleen), 5:00 (intestines), 7:00 (intestines), 11:00 (liver and gallbladder). You may feel a release in other parts of your stomach. I like to spend a lot of time in this area when I have the time. It's my favorite step in this sequence; it's very effective in softening the entire abdomen, as it releases the tension and emotional energy that accumulate when connective tissue around the organs gets tight.

Step 12
Repeat Step 5: Massage small circles around the outside of your belly button, integrating the navel pulls into your colon massage. Repeat five times. **Breathe deeply.**

Step 13
Repeat Steps 8 and 9: Scoop in front of your hip bones and rib cage.

Step 14
Massage your ascending, transverse, and descending colon again as in Step 4. Revisit any areas you feel need more attention. Make a few brush-strokes all over your stomach, and take a few cleansing breaths.

Step 15
Repeat Step 2: Stimulate the inguinal lymph nodes.

Step 16
Repeat Step 1: Stimulate the right and left supraclavicular lymphatic nodes at the base of your neck.

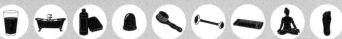

BEAUTY

Get Glowing Skin
Improve Cellulite
Slim Your Waistline

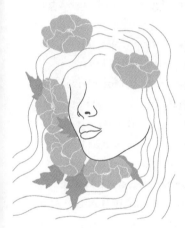

Get Glowing Skin

As your body's largest organ and its only external one, your skin is a direct reflection of your
internal state of health—physically, mentally,
and emotionally. It's how we show ourselves to
the world, and it's often the first thing we are
judged on by people, including ourselves.

The many muscles and lymph nodes in your
head and neck are constantly taking in, react-
ing to, and processing stimuli. You use your
head to think, speak, smell, sense, taste, and
experience the world. Your mouth, ears, nose,
and throat are all vulnerable to environmental toxins. If there's stagnation
under the surface of your skin as a result of clenching your jaw or staring at
a screen all day, the flow of vital nutrients and oxygen has difficulty getting
to your cells. Your lymphatic vessels' ability to remove waste can also be
hampered by muscular tension.

In order to maintain a healthy glow on the outside, you need to tend to
your inside. When toxins build up, it will show up on your skin. Alcohol and
cigarettes, for example, cause your blood vessels to dilate, leading to fluid
retention in the form of puffiness and bloating.

Imbalances in the gut can manifest as skin issues, too. An unhealthy microbiome and inflammation in the intestines, coupled with emotional stress, disrupts your skin's antimicrobial barrier; the less your skin can defend itself from bacteria, the more likely you are to have skin reactions in the form of inflammation and acne. When I have a client who complains of chronic digestive and skin problems, I always recommend that he or she take a look at his or her diet and lifestyle. That's why at the end of this sequence you will be referred to the "Abdominal Massage" sequence on page 122. I recommend alternating the "Get Glowing Skin" sequence with the "Abdominal Massage" sequence every other day for a few weeks for optimal results.

Lymphatic self-massage can also be very beneficial for people who struggle with eczema. A while back, a client who'd been suffering from eczema for more than a year came to see me when she had a red rash at the base of her neck and ears. She had been doing acupuncture and hot yoga, but her eczema had persisted. She told me that she also developed rashes that came and went in her elbow creases, in her armpits, and at the tops of her thighs—the main areas of lymph nodes. I saw her monthly for a few months, taught her self-massage, and recommended that she take a break from hot yoga as the heat might be inhibiting her lymphatic system. She was diligent with her self-care practice a few times a week and stopped turning up the heat when she did yoga. Within a few months her rash was gone and her skin tone evened out. She was truly amazed by the power of her lymphatic system in action.

In my practice, I've seen many cancer patients benefit from this sequence, as chemotherapy tends to drain the color from their faces. If you've ever noticed the skin tone of someone who has a chronic illness, the results of his or her overburdened lymph load due to fighting off a disease or processing an overwhelming amount of medications are tangible.

The lymph in the face ultimately empties to the venous angle in the subclavian vein at your collarbone. This process drains impurities from your face and down your neck, clearing out trapped bacteria, one of the root causes of breakouts. Acne is caused by the *Propionibacterium acnes* bacterium as well as hormones—which is why lymphatic massage gave my body the detox it needed and cured my zits! This sequence also affects your vagus nerve, which puts you into the parasympathetic nervous state, where your body does its best repairing and can reap the most benefits.

This sequence is a powerful double whammy. Your skin will instantly get a noticeable boost and you will activate the lymphatics in your brain, helping to cleanse plaque buildup, which, as you learned in chapter 2, has been linked to cognitive decline. Remember, you are the keeper of your body. Touch your face with love, positivity, compassion, and acceptance.

NOTE: For lots more on skin care, see chapter 5.

Step 1

Stimulate the right and left supraclavicular lymphatic nodes at the base of your neck just above your collarbone. Press your fingertips **down** into the hollows above your collarbone. Make a **J** motion as you press **lightly down** and **out** toward your shoulders. Repeat ten times.

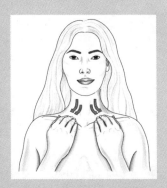

Step 2

Perform the "Neck" sequence. There are three steps.

1. Place both your palms at the base of your neck. Pulse the skin **gently** as you stroke **downward** toward your collarbone. Repeat ten times.

2. Place your hands higher so your pinky fingers rest in the groove behind your ears, your fingertips pointing diagonally toward your ears. Use your palms to stretch the skin **downward** toward your neck. Repeat five times.

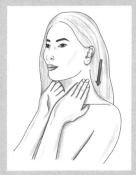 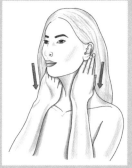 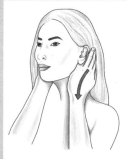

3. Make light brushstrokes from behind your ears all the way down your neck. Repeat five times. Swallow once.

Step 3

Perform the "Spock" sequence: Separate your fingers between your middle and ring fingers (Spock-like). Place your middle and index fingers behind your ears in the cartilage groove, and your ring and pinky fingers in front of your ears. **Gently** massage **back** and **downward** in a C-stroke. Repeat ten times. This stimulates both the pre- and retroauricular lymph nodes of your ears. This should be a rhythmic, nurturing movement. Swallow once.

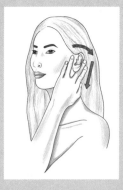

Step 4

Place your fingertips at the base of your skull, in the occipital ridge. With your fingers touching, **gently** walk your fingertips along this ridge, then glide them **down** your neck, the way a waterfall streams down a mountain. Repeat ten times.

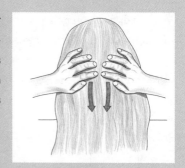

Step 5

Stimulate your shirt-collar lymphatic zone: Place your hands on top of your shoulders, your elbows pointing straight in front of you. Inhale, then drop your elbows as you exhale, keeping your fingertips on your shoulders. Repeat five times. This helps move lymphatic fluid from the back of your neck to the drains above your collarbone.

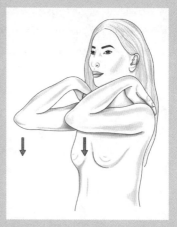

Step 6

Lightly brush your face with your fingertips from your chin to your ears, from your cheeks to your ears, from the bridge of your nose up to the middle of your forehead, then toward your ears. Then brush along your eyebrows to your ears. Repeat three times.

Step 7

Press your finger **gently** into the inner corner of each eye. Hold for three seconds. Then move your finger up to your inner eyebrows. Hold there for three seconds. Then massage along your eyebrows toward your temples. Repeat three times.

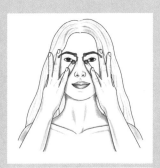

Step 8

Fan your fingertips out under your eyes. You will feel the very tops of your cheekbones here. Press **very gently** along the top line of your cheekbones toward your ears. Repeat three times.

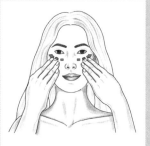

Step 9

Repeat Step 7: Press the inner corners of your eyes, then massage up to your brow bones and across your eyebrows to your temples.

Step 10

Place your right thumb underneath your right eye and your index finger on your eyebrow. **Lightly** lift your index finger as if you're "opening" the eye socket. Be as light as a feather. **Gently** walk your fingers from your eyebrows out toward your temples three times. Repeat on the left side three times.

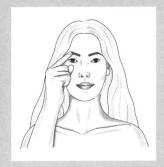

Step 11

With your fingertips, make light brushstrokes from your eyebrows up to your hairline, then smooth your skin across your forehead to your temples. This is your third eye chakra, the center of intuition. This will smooth out and unclog your furrowed brow (the Botox spot!). Repeat ten times.

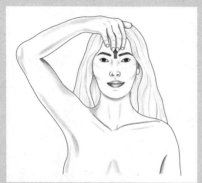 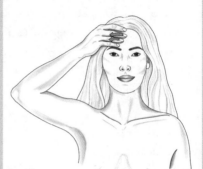

Step 12

Beginning at the inner edge of your eyebrows, **lightly** pinch along your eyebrows outward toward your temples. Repeat three times.

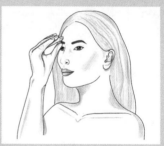

Step 13

With your fingertips, massage the crow's feet next to your eyes. Massage a figure 8 around the outsides of your eyes **very gently** ten times.

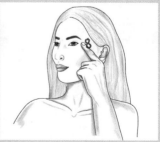

Step 14

With your fingertips, massage small C-strokes at your temples, the spot people rub when they have a headache. You can find it by opening your mouth and closing it so that your teeth touch; the muscle on the side of your forehead will move. This is a wonderful area to massage if you grind your teeth or have TMJ, but please be gentle and loving here! Repeat ten times. Swallow once.

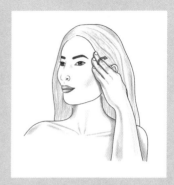

Step 15

With your fingertips, massage a wavelike pattern from your temples down to your ears, then behind your ears and down your neck to your collarbone. Swallow each time your fingers reach your neck. This will help drain the lymphatic fluid out of your face. Repeat three times.

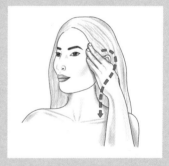

Step 16

Massage your scalp with your fingertips as if you're shampooing your hair. Massage your entire head toward the back of your scalp and down the back of your neck. I recommend massaging your scalp for about thirty seconds. This stimulates the glymphatic system in your brain.

Step 17

Place two fingertips beside each nostril where your sinuses are located. Press **lightly down** and **out**. This will drain fluid in your nasal cavity. Please be very gentle when touching the fluid just underneath your skin. Resist the urge to press too deeply. Repeat five times.

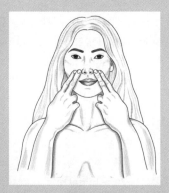

Step 18

With the pads of your fingers, **gently** tap from your nose to your cheekbones to your ears. Repeat five times. Then make light brushstrokes from your nose to your ears.

Step 19

Pinch your cheeks **lightly** from your cheekbones to your ears. Repeat five times.

Step 20

With your fingertips, massage upside-down C-strokes or rainbows on your jawline from your chin to your ears. Repeat three times.

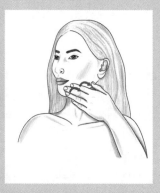

Step 21

Repeat Step 6: With your fingertips, make light brushstrokes from your chin to your ears, your cheeks to your ears, and your forehead to your ears. Repeat three times.

Step 22

Repeat Step 15: With your fingertips, massage a wavelike pattern from your temples down to your ears, then behind your ears and down your neck to your collarbone.

Step 23

Repeat Step 3, the "Spock" sequence.

Step 24

With your fingertips, massage around your lips. **Gently** massage from your lips to your ears in an upside-down C-stroke.

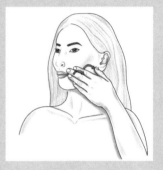

Step 25

With your right thumb and index finger, **lightly** pinch above and below your lips on the right side. **Gently** pinch all along the upper and under parts of your lip, from the center to the corner. Repeat three times. Then repeat three times on the left side.

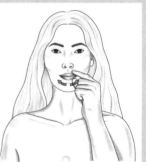

Step 26

Repeat Step 20, but this time use the heel of your hand to massage your jawline from your chin to your ears. Repeat three times.

Step 27

Repeat Step 6: **Lightly** brush your face with your fingertips from your chin to your ears, from your cheeks to your ears, from your forehead to your ears, and down the neck to your collarbone. Repeat three times.

Step 28

Repeat Step 4: Massage the occipital ridge at the base of your skull. Then make light brushstrokes behind your ear and down your neck.

Step 29

Repeat Step 3, the "Spock" sequence.

Step 30

Repeat Step 2, the "Neck" sequence.

Step 31

Repeat Step 5: Stimulate your shirt-collar lymphatic zone.

Step 32

Repeat Step 1: Stimulate the right and left supraclavicular lymphatic nodes at the base of your neck three times.

Step 33

Rub your palms together vigorously. Once they heat up, place them over your eyes. Hold them there for ten seconds as you breathe deeply. As you release your hands, press your palms into your cheekbones.

Step 34

If you have long-standing acne or are having a skin flare-up, I recommend you also do the "Abdominal Massage" sequence on page 122 to help clear up any issues in your gut that may be affecting your skin.

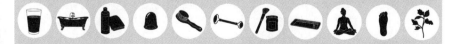

Improve Cellulite

Cellulite occurs when fat cells get trapped by bands of connective tissue close to the surface of the skin. The connective fibers under your skin break down, toxins build up, and the thin strands of skin lose elasticity, which creates bulges engorged with fat. Those fatty clusters or deposits harden and adhere to the connective tissue, or fascia. This leads to a cycle of fat accumulation, poor circulation, and skin texture changes. When the relationship between the connective tissue under the skin and fat layer is compromised, pesky dimples and lumps arise.

Cellulite is usually located in the buttocks, abdomen, hips, thighs, or arms. There are three grades:

- **Grade 1, soft.** Not painful to the touch. Commonly referred to as "orange peel" consistency. The skin can be soft and saggy looking. If you press into it with your fingertips, you will see superficial depressions. This is the easiest to affect with massage.
- **Grade 2, moderate.** This stage signifies a combination of fluid retention (edema) and connective tissue adhering to the skin. Insufficient circulation can lead to fatty deposits building up in the tissues underneath the skin. If you press into it with your fingertips, the skin depressions are deeper and may be painful to the touch.
- **Grade 3, severe.** Typically chronic, this cellulite can be hard and painful to the touch. This is often referred to as a "mattress" appearance. Fluid movement under the skin is severely limited. When cellulite becomes fibrotic, it takes longer to treat.

Cellulite can appear no matter how much or how little you weigh or how much your weight fluctuates. It can also be caused by hormonal swings, pregnancy, hereditary factors, or stress—which can cause the surrounding connective tissue and muscles to constrict, disrupting circulation and preventing proper elimination—as well as by poor digestion. The amount of cellulite you have may also fluctuate depending on your diet and exercise regimen.

Some people are plagued with a condition called **lipedema** that doesn't change much even when they eat well and exercise regularly. Lipedema is believed to be linked to a hereditary gene because it tends to run in the family. Those with this condition are often dismissed by doctors, and their condition is neither validated nor understood. There's an entire field of lymphedema therapy devoted to strategies for lipedema clients suffering from persistent fat deposits in the skin. If that's you, see Resources, page 316. I encourage you to work with a lymphedema therapist who specializes in lipedema.

Saggy skin, dimples, and uncomfortable weight gain are all signs of stagnant lymphatic fluid. This sequence can help the appearance of cellulite over time and bring back healthy micro blood circulation to improve venous circulation and lymphatic circulation. It's not an immediate fix. For many, the appearance of cellulite is frustrating, though it is largely a fact of life: some 80 to 90 percent of women will experience it to some degree. Though self-massage will help diminish the appearance of cellulite, it can also promote better lymph flow to the affected areas.

Because fat is stored in the tissues and lymphatic system, by focusing on flushing trapped toxins, you can aid in detoxifying the area, which will improve your skin tone. In addition to lymphatic treatments, dry-brush daily and do lymphatic cupping (see "How to Do Lymphatic Cupping" on page 292). Reducing your intake of dairy products and gluten, increasing your water and vegetable intake, and exercising regularly will all help support this detoxification as well. Targeted isometric strength training is particularly beneficial, especially around the abdomen, legs, and butt. It will tighten your muscles and create the extra oxygen consumption needed to use up that fat. I also love using scrubs and oils containing caffeine; caffeine can temporarily dehydrate fat cells, but the superficial skin effects last for only a few hours.

This sequence clears the lymph nodes and pathways to eliminate toxins first, then focuses on decongesting the stubborn fatty tissue with deeper pressure using hand-rolling and finger-folding techniques to target stubborn spots and free blockages. Combine this sequence with the "Achy Limbs: Legs" sequence on page 223 for maximum impact.

NOTE: You may want to use some lymphatic leg-firming cellulite oil for this sequence. Look for one containing caffeine and/or linseed oil, which can be found in most stores where skin care products are sold.

Step 1

Sit in a comfortable position. Begin by doing some deep abdominal breathing. This will increase your lymphatic absorption and transportation rate. Place your hands on your abdomen. Take a deep breath into your abdomen, expanding your abdomen into your hands as if you're blowing up a balloon. As you exhale, relax your abdomen. Repeat ten times.

Step 2

Place one hand on your abdomen and the other over your heart. Visualize your thoracic duct, which runs from your abdomen to your heart. When you inhale, visualize the trunk of a tree rising up your midline from your navel, its branches extending through your lungs and into your heart. As you exhale, visualize the leaves of the tree swaying in the wind. Repeat ten times.

Step 3

Stimulate your inguinal lymph nodes: Two hand placements. Place your hand on top of your inner thigh. Massage C-strokes **upward** to the crease at the top of your thigh. Repeat ten times. Repeat on your outer thigh.

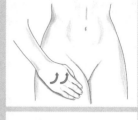

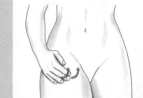

Step 4

Lift each leg six times. This movement stimulates your inguinal lymph nodes.

Step 5

Massage your upper thigh. You can use one or both hands.

1. Outer thigh: Massage overlapping C-strokes from the outside of your knee **upward** toward the inguinal lymph nodes along the outer side of your thigh. Repeat ten times.
2. Center thigh: Massage overlapping C-strokes from the center of your knee **up** the middle of your leg to your inguinal lymph nodes. Repeat ten times.
3. Inner thigh: Massage overlapping C-strokes from the inside of your knee **upward** to the top of your inner thigh. Repeat ten times.

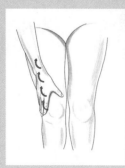
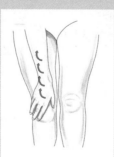
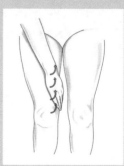

4. Back of the thigh: Bend your leg so
   you can reach underneath your thigh.
   With both hands, sweep the fluid from
   your hamstrings to the front of your
   leg into your inguinal lymph nodes.
   Repeat ten times. Pump your inguinal
   lymph nodes again three times.

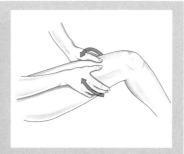

Step 6

Repeat Step 5 on your opposite upper thigh.

Step 7

Massage your knee.

1. Place the palm of your hand under
   your knee. Pump upward directly
   into the back of your knee; you have
   lymph nodes here (the popliteal
   fossa). Repeat ten times.

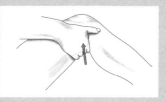

2. Place both hands on each side of
   your kneecap. Grab the skin on
   both sides of your knee, and make
   C-strokes **upward**. Repeat ten
   times.

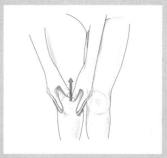

3. Place your hand on top of your kneecap. Stroke your skin **up** and **over** your knee. Repeat ten times.

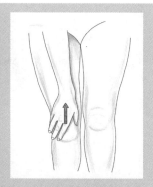

Step 8

Repeat Step 7 on your opposite knee.

Now that you have moved stagnant lymph from the area, you can perform the following strokes specific to cellulite reduction. These strokes can be deeper than your usual lymph massage strokes as you are now focusing on the fat layer.

Step 9

Find an area of concentrated cellulite. Spread a small amount of cellulite-targeting oil over the area. Next, pinch a small area of skin between your fingertips. With more pressure than in typical lymphatic self-massage, grab and lift your skin, then roll the skin up **toward** your inguinal lymph nodes. This is the secret technique of cellulite machines—they lift and roll the skin. Repeat ten times. Find another area of cellulite close by and continue lifting and rolling toward your inguinal lymph nodes.

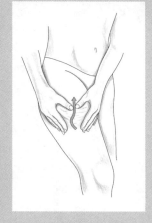

Step 10

Do a knuckle massage: With a loose fist over a patch of cellulite, roll over the skin with your knuckles in overlapping C-strokes toward your inguinal lymph nodes. Repeat ten times.

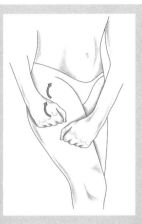

Step 11

Knead the skin with your hands in three vertical lines. Repeat each line ten times as if you are kneading dough. Cellulite in women is arranged vertically, so work vertically toward your inguinal lymph nodes.

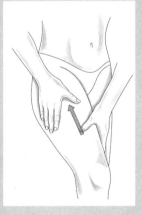

Step 12

Do finger spirals: With your thumb or fingers over a smaller area, concentrate on smoothing out your skin as you would folds from a crumpled piece of paper. Make smaller tight, short strokes now. This might be more tender or painful, as you are using slightly more pressure than in other sequences as you work on breaking up fat deposits. Take inventory of the texture and color of your skin. You don't want to become bruised. As you bring more blood to the area, it may change the color of your skin temporarily. Slow down and rest for a moment to let your skin return to normal if this persists.

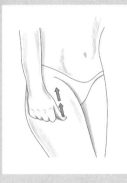

Step 13
Repeat Step 5: Massage your upper thigh. Repeat on the opposite upper thigh.

Step 14
Repeat Step 7: Massage under your knee, then over the knee, then do the same on your opposite knee. Massage the sides of your knee up to your thigh.

Step 15
Repeat Step 3: Stimulate your inguinal lymph nodes.

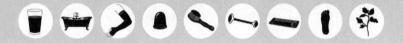

Slim Your Waistline

The secret of a slimmer waistline is what I like to call a "triple threat": diet, massage, and exercise. As you learned in chapters 1 and 2, the lymphatic system helps maintain the fluid balance in the body and absorbs excess fat in the gut. Lymphatic massage is famous for helping people achieve a slimmer waistline. To keep excess weight off, you'll need to do some exercises that will help increase your lymphatic circulation. You can find a list of them beginning on page 308. It's also essential to keep yourself hydrated to encourage transportation of lymphatic debris through its vasculature. You'll find lists of foods to eat and foods to avoid beginning on page 272 that will help you maintain a slimmer stomach.

Finally, I recommend that you massage your abdomen regularly, at least three or four times a week. Increasing the peristalsis of your internal organs will help you eliminate congested waste, break up tight connective tissue, and keep your bowel movements regular. That's the lymphatic way to lose some inches and keep it off.

I also recommend the "Abdominal Massage" sequence on page 122.

YOUR INTERNAL LANDSCAPE

Calm Anxiety
Energy and Mental Clarity
Hangover Remedy
Heart and Lung Opener
Good Sleep

Calm Anxiety

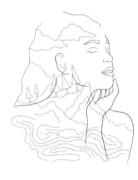

Many of us experience some degree of anxiety. Our world is filled with situations and stressors we are constantly trying to manage, and the value placed on productivity and achievement makes many people feel chronically anxious about whether or not they are "doing enough." Research has shown that attending to the 24/7 news cycle—made even worse by social media—is taking an additional toll on our mental health.

In my practice, I see every day how anxiety manifests itself in the body and causes inflammation. I encourage you to take inventory of the internal and external forces in your life that make you feel anxious. What things can you let go of that are causing you unnecessary stress and worry? Taking the time to do an honest self-assessment of the pressures that are weighing on you is as important to mitigating your anxiety as self-massage. I also recommend trying the meditation technique described on page 303, as meditation is a proven way to help calm the body and reduce anxiety.

One reason anxiety impacts us physiologically is that our breathing changes dramatically when we are under stress. When we're nervous or uncomfortable, we tend to hold our breath or take shallow breaths. Without your realizing it, tension gets trapped in your shoulders or creates tightness in your chest, rib cage, and diaphragm, which can impact your lungs and even your digestion. Similarly, your throat can feel as though it's closing, leading to a temporary inability to speak up or express yourself. This can create a crippling loop of anxiety. Because breathing is integral to pumping lymph, this massage sequence includes abdominal breathing to open the respiratory pathways along your sternum and bring more oxygen into your lungs.

Your solar plexus, the home of the third chakra (self-esteem and personal power), which is located near the thymus, the lymphoid organ that matures and produces fighter T cells that guard against disease, will also play a role in this sequence. This sequence will stimulate lymphatic circulation, unlock congestion, alleviate anxiety, calm your central nervous system, and get you out of your head and into your heart.

Step 1

Begin by sitting so you're comfortable. Stimulate the right and left supraclavicular lymphatic nodes at the base of your neck. The right and left lymphatic nodes are located just above your collarbone. Press your fingertips **down** into the hollows above your collarbone. Make a **J** motion as you press **lightly down** and **out** toward your shoulders. Repeat ten times.

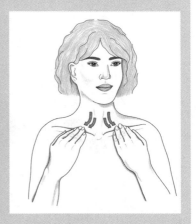

Step 2

Stimulate the axillary lymph nodes in your armpits. There are three steps:

1. Place your hand inside your armpit, your index finger resting **gently** in the groove of your armpit. Pulse **upward** into your armpit. Repeat ten times.
2. Move your hand **down** the side of your torso. This region contains breast tissue, which is essential to drain. With the palm of your hand, make C-strokes from the side of your torso **upward** into your armpit. Repeat ten times.
3. Lift your arm and place your hand into your armpit. Pump **downward** over your armpit ten times. Release your arm.

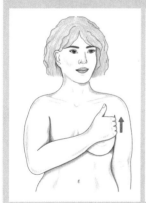
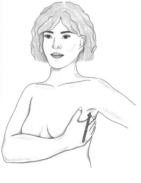
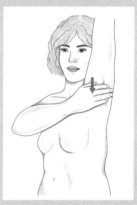

Step 3
Repeat Step 2 on your opposite armpit.

Step 4
Stimulate your shirt-collar lymphatic zone: Place your hands on top of your shoulders, your elbows pointing straight in front of you. Inhale, then drop your elbows as you exhale, keeping your fingertips on your shoulders. Repeat five times. This helps move lymphatic fluid from the back of your neck to the drains above your collarbone. It also helps relax your trapezius muscle, which gets tight with anxiety and worry.

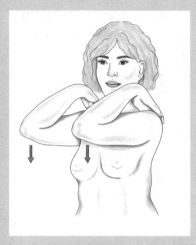

Step 5
Place the palm of your right hand above your left breast, fingertips facing your armpit. **Gently** massage C-strokes over the top of your breast toward your left armpit. Repeat five times.

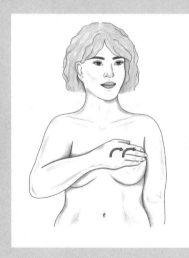

Step 6
Repeat on the right side.

Step 7

Place your palm in the center of your chest, over your breastbone. Massage upside-down C-strokes as if you're drawing a rainbow over your heart and lungs. Take a slow, deep breath into your hand. Count to three on each inhale, and count backward from three to one as you exhale. With each inhale, feel your chest rise into your hand. As you exhale, allow your chest to relax and soften. Repeat at least three times, but feel free to do this step as many times as needed to release tension.

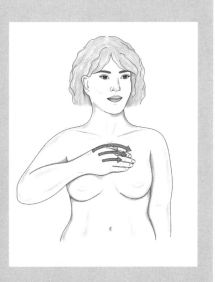

Step 8

Place the fingertips of both hands along your sternum. The grooves here are near your intercostal muscles, which help you to breathe. **Very gently**, press **in** and **out** ten times. As you are working only on the fluid layer, resist the urge to press deeply.

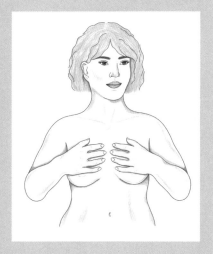

Step 9

Repeat Step 7: Place your palm in the center of your chest, over your breastbone. Massage rainbows over your chest as you take five deep breaths. Rock your body back and forth. This rocking motion mimics the undulating wavelike rhythm of lymphatic drainage, which soothes your entire state of being. Repeat five times.

Step 10

Repeat Steps 5 and 6: Massage C-strokes over each breast toward your armpits.

Step 11

Do abdominal breathing: Place your hands on your abdomen. Take a deep breath into your abdomen. With each inhale, expand your abdomen into your hands like a balloon. As you exhale, let your abdomen relax. Repeat five times. This will propel lymph from the lower half of your body and engage your rest-and-digest parasympathetic nervous system, where healing occurs.

Step 12

Place one hand on your abdomen and the other hand over your heart. Imagine there are disks of energy running from your belly to your heart. As you inhale, visualize the color orange at your second chakra, just below your navel. Move your breath higher through your lungs to your third chakra and envision the color yellow, like a radiant sun. When your breath reaches your heart, the fourth chakra, imagine the color bright green in your chest. As you exhale, allow your abdomen to relax. Repeat three times. This is the pathway that your thoracic duct moves to return lymphatic fluid to your blood circulation. This potent breath can be done anytime you need to release anxiety and access a calmer state of being.

Step 13
With one hand still over your heart and the other on your abdomen, breathe deeply into your abdomen as you massage C-strokes over your heart. Say "Heeeeee" out loud as you exhale. This sound helps balance the energy centers of the body from the lower navel to the heart. Repeat five times.

Step 14
Lightly tap your fingertips over your sternum. Visualize the sound of the thumping down into your cells. This is where your T cell–maturing thymus is located, above your heart. The thymus stores immature white blood cells and gets them ready to become active T cells that mount an immune response to destroy infected and nefarious cells. As you tap your chest, imagine all the benefits of your thymus.

Step 15
Repeat Steps 2 and 3: Stimulate the axillary lymph nodes in your armpits three times.

Step 16
Repeat Step 4: Stimulate your shirt-collar lymphatic zone.

Step 17
Stretch your neck to release tension. Looking forward, tilt your right ear toward your shoulder. Holding it there, breathe in and out three times. Repeat on the left side.

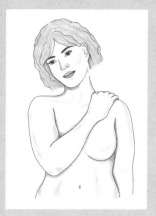

Step 18

Circle your head in each direction three times. (If you are prone to getting dizzy or suffering from vertigo, skip this step.)

Step 19

Lift your shoulders and squeeze them up toward your ears. Hold for three seconds, breathing in and out. Release your shoulders. Repeat three times.

Step 20

Make light brushstrokes on your face from your cheeks to your ears, from your chin to your ears, from the bridge of your nose up to your forehead, and from your forehead to your ears. Repeat three times.

Step 21

Massage your scalp with your fingertips as if you're shampooing your hair for as long as it takes to sing "Happy Birthday."

Step 22

Place your fingertips at the base of your skull, in the occipital ridge. With your fingers touching, **gently** walk your fingertips along this ridge, then glide them **down** your neck the way a waterfall streams down a mountain. Repeat ten times.

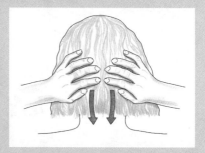

Step 23

Make light brushstrokes down the front of your neck to your right and left lymphatic nodes at the collarbones. Repeat five times. Swallow twice.

Step 24

Rub your palms together vigorously. Once they heat up, place them over your eyes. Hold them there for a few seconds as you breathe deeply. Imagine the color violet from the crown of your head down to your toes. Relax your forehead, eyes, face, and throat. As you open your eyes, press the heels of your hands along your cheekbones toward your ears.

Step 25

Repeat Step 4: Stimulate your shirt-collar lymphatic zone.

Step 26

Repeat Steps 2 and 3: Stimulate the axillary lymph nodes in your armpits three times.

Step 27

Repeat Step 1: Stimulate the right and left supraclavicular lymphatic nodes at the base of your neck.

Step 28

Swallow twice. Place your hands into your lap and smile. Scan your body to see how you feel.

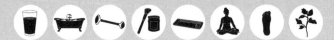

Energy and Mental Clarity

Energy

When clients come in for a session, I always inquire how they're feeling and ask them to rate their energy level from one to ten. All too often, the number they name is less than five—they're feeling burned out and run-down. Some feel too tired to exercise—or even too tired to *think* about exercising, even though they know it will give them more energy.

What is energy, and where do we feel it? Do you recognize it when you have it or only when you don't? I can tell you that when you work on your lymph, your energy will change. People notice it immediately. Many of my clients report that they feel "lighter" and "clearer," and have less pain. Sometimes they experience sensations associated with detoxification, similar to the way you might feel on day three of a cleanse—a little light-headed and very tired. This is a common feeling that can occur when you begin to move trapped waste out of your tissues.

This series provides a combination of short exercises designed to move stagnant energy and increase your lymphatic flow. If you've ever had acu-puncture, you know that Chinese medicine is based on the concept of *chi*, life energy that flows through certain meridians in your body. Acu-puncture needles inserted at various meridian points can free up this *chi*, much as lymphatic self-massage can free toxic buildup in your interstitial spaces. This sequence moves stagnant energy through your body, clean-ing out the gunk and debris that is making you feel sluggish and inhibiting you from feeling your best.

The quickest way to get more energy is to stimulate all your drains—your lymph node regions—in your neck, armpit, thymus, belly, and groin. This sequence incorporates some movements from qigong (similar to tai chi, with slow, concentrated movements and an emphasis on breathing) and yoga to activate the hinges of your body where your lymph nodes cluster, serving as a full toxin flush to improve your energy and restore mental clarity.

Mental Clarity

Have you ever forgotten about an important meeting or phone call even though it was on your calendar? Or struggled to recall the details of a conversation? Misplaced your keys? Brain fog can interfere with your life in such small ways, and it can also cloud your judgment, making it difficult to make decisions or know the right path to take.

It's often challenging to pinpoint the cause of brain fog, as it can stem from poor diet, lack of sleep, medications, hormonal imbalances, or mental health factors. If you've ever referred to yourself as having "mommy brain," "chemo brain," "lack-of-sleep brain," "no-coffee brain," "multitasking brain," "selective listening brain," or "COVID-brain," this sequence is for you.

The glymphatic pathways that help clear drainage in the brain, as discussed in chapter 2, are stimulated in this sequence to help move out the stagnation that interferes with thinking clearly and feeling vibrant. Because this sequence focuses on the head, neck, jaw, and breath, you will create a systemic lymphatic wave to help release tension in your face and encourage fluid absorption and recirculation.

Step 1

From a comfortable seated or standing position, stimulate the right and left supraclavicular lymphatic nodes at the base of your neck just above your collarbone. Press your fingertips **down** into the hollows above your collarbone. Make a J motion as you press **lightly down** and **out** toward your shoulders. Repeat ten times.

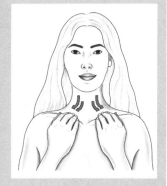

Step 2

Perform the "Neck" sequence. There are three steps.

1. Place both your palms at the base of your neck. Pulse the skin **gently** as you stroke **downward** toward your collarbone. Repeat ten times.
2. Place your hands higher so your pinky fingers rest in the groove behind your ears, your fingertips pointing diagonally toward your ears. Use your palms to stretch the skin **downward** toward your neck. Repeat five times.
3. Make light brushstrokes from behind your ears all the way down your neck. Repeat five times. Swallow once.

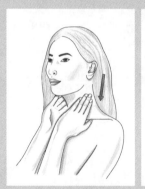 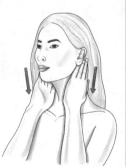 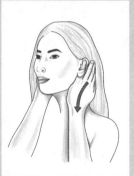

Step 3

Perform the "Spock" sequence: Separate your fingers between your middle and ring fingers (Spock-like). Place your middle and index fingers behind your ears in the cartilage groove and your ring and pinky fingers in front of your ears. **Gently** massage **back** and **downward** in a C-stroke. Repeat ten times. This stimulates both the pre- and retroauricular lymph nodes of your ears. This should be a rhythmic, nurturing movement. Swallow once.

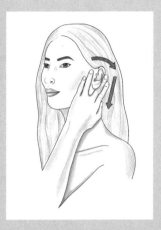

Step 4

Make light brushstrokes on your face from your chin to your ears, from your cheeks to your ears, and from your forehead to your ears.

Step 5

Place your fingertips at the base of your skull, in the occipital ridge. With your fingers touching, **gently** walk your fingertips along this ridge, then glide them **down** your neck, the way a waterfall streams down a mountain. Repeat ten times.

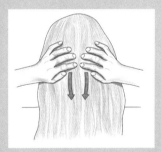

Step 6

Massage your scalp with your fingertips as if you're shampooing your hair. Massage your entire head toward the back of your scalp and down the back of your neck. This stimulates the glymphatic system in your brain.

Step 7

Stimulate your shirt-collar lymphatic zone: Place your hands on top of your shoulders, your elbows pointing straight in front of you. Inhale, then drop your elbows as you exhale, keeping your fingertips on your shoulders. Repeat five times. This helps move lymphatic fluid from the back of your neck to the drains above your collarbone.

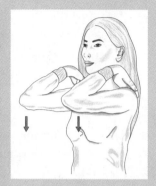

Step 8

Stimulate the axillary nodes. Place your hand inside your armpit, your index finger resting gently in the groove of your armpit. Pulse **upward** into your armpit. Repeat ten times.

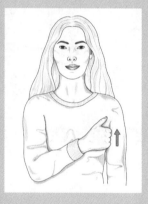

Step 9

Repeat Step 8 on your opposite armpit.

Step 10

Do a thymus tap: Place the palm of one hand on your chest, and with your fingertips **lightly** tap the thymus area on your sternum. Some of your breast fluid drains into the mammary chain of lymph nodes here. This is also where your active T cells, which fight infection, mature. Repeat ten times.

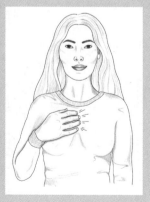

Step 11

Do abdominal breathing: Place your hands on your abdomen. As you inhale, expand your abdomen into your hands like a balloon. As you exhale, let your abdomen relax. Repeat five times. This stimulates the cisterna chyli and thoracic duct to move lymph from the lower half of your body.

Step 12

Stimulate the inguinal lymph nodes: Place your hand on the top of your inner right thigh in the thigh crease. This is where your inguinal lymph nodes are located. Lift your leg six times. Massage C-strokes **upward** into the crease of your thigh. Repeat five times.

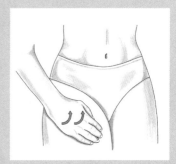

Step 13

Repeat Step 12 on your opposite thigh.

Step 14

If you've been seated, stand up. Stretch your neck, tilting your right ear toward your shoulder. Breathe deeply in and out as you hold the stretch for ten seconds before you release. Repeat on the left side. Repeat twice. This is a simple way to clear some tension in your throat chakra.

Step 15

Make five neck circles slowly in each direction. If you are prone to vertigo, skip this step.

Step 16

Do shoulder lifts: Lift your shoulders toward your ears. Inhale, hold your breath for three seconds, then exhale and relax your shoulders. Repeat five times.

Step 17

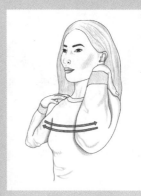

Do a twist rotation: Place your hands on top of your shoulders. As you breathe, twist your torso from side to side, keeping your hands on your shoulders. Repeat ten times. This is a nice way to get some energy flowing through your heart and solar plexus chakras.

Step 18

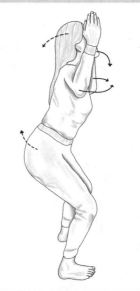

Bend your knees slightly. Bring your elbows together in front of your face. If you can't get your elbows to touch, it's okay if they are slightly separated. With your elbows bent, inhale and look up while you stretch your arms as wide as you can to the sides, and stick your butt out behind you. Exhale and curl your elbows, hips, and butt back into the center of your body, and look down toward your elbows. Gradually increase your speed so you are moving back and forth quickly. (This is similar to the cat/cow yoga pose, only you're standing up.) Repeat twenty times quickly. This brings movement into your pelvic floor and root chakra.

Step 19

With loose arms, twist your entire body from side to side like Wonder Woman. Allow your hands to hit the back of your body at your shoulder level, waist level, and hip level. Repeat twenty times.

Step 20

Place your hands on your hips. Make hip circles ten times in each direction.

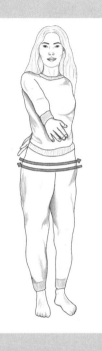

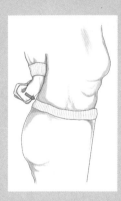

Step 21

Bend your knees and hold your hands in loose fists. Using the backs of your hands, **lightly** tap your lower back at your kidneys. This will stimulate and wake up your kidneys and adrenals. Repeat twenty times.

Step 22

Place your hands on your knees. Make circles with your knees in each direction ten times.

Step 23

Stand tall. Lift your arms out to the sides and over your head toward the sky, gathering new energy and life force all the way up until your palms touch. Then bring your hands to your heart in prayer or *namaste* position. Repeat five times.

Step 24

Rub your palms together vigorously. Once they heat up, place them over your eyes as you breathe deeply. As you release your hands, press your palms into your cheekbones.

Step 25

Smile. Take a deep breath in, and, as you exhale, smile and say "Ha" as though you're laughing. Do this at least five times. This will activate your internal organs, so feel free to laugh for as long as you want!

NOTE: When I'm short on time, I often do just the movement portion of this sequence. It's okay to skip the opening of drains if you're pressed for time. But if you have time to do the entire sequence, you will notice a major shift in your energy level and an improvement in your mental clarity.

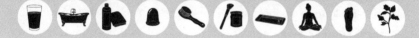

Hangover Remedy

It happens. Many articles have been written and folklore recipes handed down about how best to deal with a hangover. Lymphatic self-massage can be extremely helpful in accelerating the detoxification process, because, after all, it's your lymphatic system's job to clear out excess toxins from your tissues.

Remember that detoxifying is at the root of eliminating a hangover. How many times have you heard that one of the best ways to get rid of a hangover is to sweat? That's because sweating helps flush toxins from your body and increase your blood flow.

In addition, when you drink too much alcohol, it can limit your stomach's ability to destroy harmful bacteria there, allowing it to enter your upper small intestine. Lymphatically, that can impair the mucus cells that protect your stomach wall from being damaged by acid and digestive enzymes, causing inflammation. This is a reason why your stomach becomes bloated after too many glasses of wine or martinis.

I have to admit I've done this sequence on myself many times—and it really works. It's a blend of the "Earache" sequence on page 90 and the "Headache" sequence on page 99 with a short abdominal massage for good measure. It's specifically designed to aid your recovery, get rid of your headache, quell inflammation, restore your vibrancy, and make you feel brighter. Be sure to drink a lot of water afterward. An Epsom salt bath will also help draw out toxins and speed your recovery.

Sometimes I start this sequence immediately after drinking a glass of wine during a dinner party or before I go to bed. Don't fret if you're not that organized; you can still use this sequence the next day. Because the liver is involved in processing alcohol and is also susceptible to inflammation with prolonged alcohol use, I recommend you also try the "Abdominal Massage" sequence on page 122 and spend some time stimulating your liver to release the toxic load.

Step 1

Stimulate the right and left supraclavicular lymphatic nodes at the base of your neck just above your collarbone. Press your fingertips **down** into the hollows above your collarbone. Make a **J** motion as you press **lightly down** and **out** toward your shoulders. Repeat ten times.

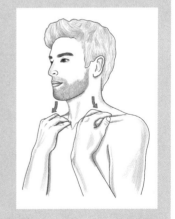

Step 2

Perform the "Neck" sequence. There are three steps:

1. Place both your palms at the base of your neck. Pulse the skin **gently** as you stroke **downward** toward your collarbone. Repeat ten times.

2. Place your hands higher so your pinky fingers rest in the groove behind your ears, your fingertips pointing diagonally toward your ears. Use your palms to stretch the skin **downward** toward your neck. Repeat five times.

3. Make light brushstrokes from behind your ears all the way down your neck. Repeat five times. Swallow once.

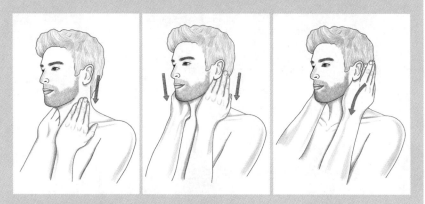

Step 3

Perform the "Spock" sequence: Separate your fingers between your middle and ring fingers (Spock-like). Place your middle and index fingers behind your ears in the cartilage groove, and your ring and pinky fingers in front of your ears. **Gently** massage **back** and **downward** in a C-stroke. Repeat ten times. This stimulates both the pre- and retroauricular lymph nodes of your ears. This should be a rhythmic, nurturing movement. Swallow once.

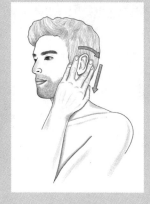

Step 4

Place your fingertips at the base of your skull, in the occipital ridge. With your fingers touching, **gently** walk your fingertips along this ridge, then glide them **down** your neck, the way a waterfall streams down a mountain. Repeat ten times.

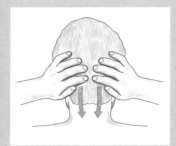

Step 5

Stimulate your shirt-collar lymphatic zone: Place your hands on top of your shoulders, your elbows pointing straight in front of you. Inhale, then drop your elbows as you exhale, keeping your fingertips on your shoulders. Repeat five times. This helps move lymphatic fluid from the back of your neck to the drains above your collarbone.

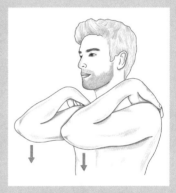

Step 6

Lightly brush your face with your fingers from your chin to your ears, from your cheeks to your ears, and from the bridge of your nose up to your forehead, then to your ears. Repeat three times.

Step 7

Massage your scalp with your fingertips as if you're shampooing your hair. Massage your entire head toward the back of your scalp and down the back of your neck. This stimulates the glymphatic system in your brain.

Step 8

Draw rainbows on your scalp. There are three steps:

1. Place your right hand on top of your head at the center of your scalp. Make "rainbows" with the heel of your hand down the right side of your scalp to move the fluid toward the back of your neck. Stop just behind your right ear. Repeat five times. Repeat on the left side five times.

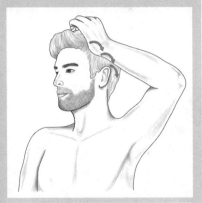

2. Place your right hand a little farther down on your scalp and closer to your ear. Make "rainbows" with the heel of your hand **downward** toward the back of your neck. Repeat five times. Repeat on the left side five times.

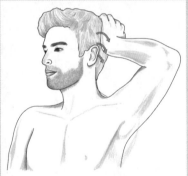

3. Place both hands on the top of your head, closer to the occiput at the base of your skull. With the heels of your hands, make C-strokes all the way down the back of your neck. Repeat five times.

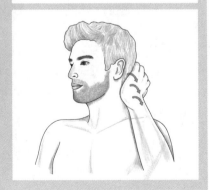

Step 9
Place your hands behind your ears, your pinky fingers resting in the carti-lage groove. **Gently** glide the heels of your hands **downward** in a C-stroke. Repeat ten times.

Step 10
Repeat Step 3, the "Spock" sequence.

Step 11
Lightly brush your forehead from the center to your ears, from your hair-line to your ears, and from your neck down to your collarbone. Repeat three times.

Step 12
Repeat Step 1: Stimulate the right and left supraclavicular lymphatic nodes at the base of your neck. Swallow once.

Step 13
Do ear pulls:

1. With your right index finger and thumb, **gently** stretch the cartilage inside your earlobe **downward** and **outward** toward the back of your head. Hold for ten seconds, breathing deeply. Release your ear, open and close your mouth twice, and swallow once.

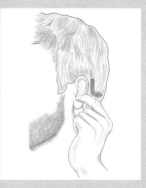

2. Move your index finger and thumb to another spot inside your earlobe. **Gently**

stretch the lobe **downward** and **outward**, toward the back of your head. Hold for ten seconds, breathing deeply. Release your earlobe, open and close your mouth twice, and swallow once.

3. Continue working all along your earlobe up to the very top of your ear. **Gently** stretch the cartilage in each place **outward** toward the back of your scalp, and hold for ten seconds. (If you are wearing earrings, be mindful to avoid them.)

Step 14
Repeat Step 13 on your left ear.

Step 15
Repeat Step 8: Draw rainbows on your scalp.

Step 16
Lightly brush your forehead from the center to your ears, from your eyebrows to your ears, from your cheeks to your ears, from your chin to your ears, from your ears down your neck, and each side of your head down the back of your neck.

Step 17
Repeat Step 5: Stimulate your shirt-collar lymphatic zone.

Step 18
Repeat Step 1: Stimulate the right and left supraclavicular lymphatic nodes at the base of your neck. Swallow once.

Step 19

Do an abdominal massage. This will help detox your liver and move out any stored tension in your abdomen. With the palm of one hand, make overlapping circles all around your colon: up the right side, across your abdomen, and down your left side. Make circles under your navel toward your left hip. Allow your strokes 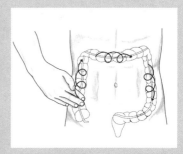 to be nourishing and simple. Use as much of your palm and fingers as possible. Circle your abdomen at least ten times.

Step 20

Massage small circles around the circumference of your belly button. You can use a little more pressure here, as this is where your deeper network of lymph resides. If you find some tight areas, spend some time nourishing yourself there.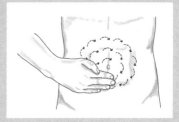

Step 21

Repeat Step 19: Do an abdominal massage, kneading your belly happily like a purring cat. Revisit any areas needing more attention.

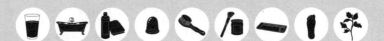

Heart and Lung Opener

Your lungs are beautiful cone-shaped organs that rest on either side of your heart. Connected to your trachea, they span from just below your collarbone to your sixth rib. Your bronchial and pulmonary lymph nodes receive lymphatic fluid from your lungs. Deep diaphragmatic breathing stimulates your thoracic duct, which moves lymph from your lower extremities and abdomen back up toward your heart. Deep breathing also increases your lung capacity and has a positive effect on your parasympathetic rest-and-digest response. Most major surgeries for which anesthesia is administered require that patients show stable lung capacity, as measured with an oxygen pulse oximeter, prior to being discharged from the hospital. Maintaining good respiratory health will enable you to defend yourself against infections, reoxygenate your cells, and expel carbon dioxide. Your lumbar lymph nodes are located between the diaphragm and the pelvis, which drain pelvic organs and the abdominal wall.

Since the COVID-19 pandemic began, more attention has been paid to the importance of maintaining healthy lung function. Some COVID-19 survivors have experienced significant scarring in their lungs; others infected were often asymptomatic and unaware that their oxygen levels were dangerously low until the virus had caused severe lung damage; and those who had previously received radiation in the chest area (from cancer treatment) or had preexisting lung disease turned out to be at greater risk of developing long-term damage. On the other hand, people who were able to do deep breathing found that it helped aid their recovery.

Drainage of the lungs is complex, as you read in chapter 2. In this sequence you will cultivate a deep breathing practice to build your lung capacity so as to increase your oxygen levels and support and maintain the intrinsic muscle movements that pump your lymph. You will also be stimulating several sets of lymph nodes that activate the pathways involved in draining your lungs of excess waste surrounding the pleura (the fluid sacs around the lungs) and the layer that cushions the respiratory tract, which reduces the friction between the lungs, rib cage, and chest cavity. The more mobility you encourage in your chest, the less fluid will build up and the more you will alleviate inflammation, adhesions, and stagnation.

Because my mother had lung cancer, it's always been a top priority of mine to give my lungs some extra TLC—and that includes tending to the emotional trauma from that loss. I often look to the Chinese Five-Element Theory as well as yoga to balance my chakras when I feel overwhelmed by my emotions. Traditional Chinese medicine (TCM) offers a way to move through physical and emotional blocks, and diaphragmatic breathing is a cornerstone of that work. I see it as the intersection of TCM and lymphatic health. The breath work down-regulates the active nervous system and promotes a healing state. In TCM, the lungs are associated with sadness and grief. Whenever I'm feeling melancholy or it's the anniversary of my mother's passing or her birthday, I do the "Heart and Lung Opener" sequence on page 175 (and I watch a funny movie, because laughter is great for moving the diaphragm). It opens the heart chakra, where breath gets trapped and affects posture. I find with my clients, too, that when you acknowledge your feelings and give yourself the space to experience and move through them, the painful associations are less likely to take root in your body.

NOTE: Do not perform this sequence if you currently have an untreated lung infection. For optimal results, avoid smoking nicotine-containing products and limit vaping.

Step 1

Stimulate the right and left supraclavicular lymphatic nodes at the base of your neck just above your collarbone. Press your fingertips **down** into the hollows above your collarbone. Make a **J** motion as you press **lightly down** and **out** toward your shoulders. Repeat ten times.

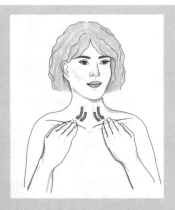

Step 2

Perform the "Neck" sequence. There are three steps:

1. Place both your palms at the base of your neck. Pulse the skin **gently** as you stroke **downward** toward your collarbone. Repeat ten times.
2. Place your hands higher so your pinky fingers rest in the groove behind your ears, your fingertips pointing diagonally toward your ears. Use your palms to stretch the skin **downward** toward your neck. Repeat five times.
3. Make light brushstrokes from behind your ears all the way down your neck. Repeat five times. Swallow once.

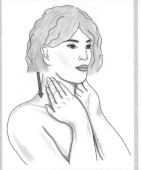
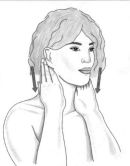
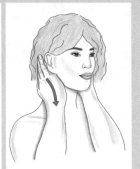

Step 3

Stimulate the axillary lymph nodes in your armpits. There are three steps:

1. Place your hand inside your armpit, your index finger resting **gently** in the groove of your armpit. Pulse **upward** into your armpit. Repeat ten times.
2. Move your hand **down** the side of your torso. This region contains breast tissue, which is essential to drain. With the palm of your hand, make C-strokes **up** the side of your torso into your armpit. Repeat ten times.
3. Lift your arm and place your hand into your armpit. Pump **downward** over your armpit ten times. Release your arm.

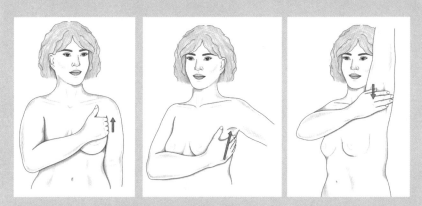

Step 4

Repeat Step 3 on your opposite armpit.

Step 5

Make large circles with your arms backward and forward to create mobility around your chest. Repeat ten times each side.

Step 6

Some of your lymphatic fluid drains to the intercostal nodes in your sternum in your torso cavity. Stimulating the nodes at your sternum creates a vacuum effect. Place your fingertips on your chest in the intercostal spaces along your sternum. You will feel the indents of your rib cage. **Very gently**, press **in** and **out** along the grooves of your intercostals. Inhale and exhale deeply. This will help pump air out of your lungs.

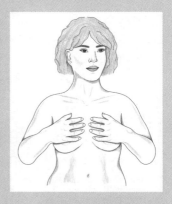

Focus on the tissue, not the muscles. You don't want to press deeply, as your skin is thin here and you are working only on the fluid layer. This is where your heart chakra lies; treat it with acceptance, self-love, and tenderness. Repeat twenty times.

Step 7

Draw rainbows over your chest: Place the palm of one hand in the center of your chest, over your breastbone. Take a slow, deep breath, and feel your chest rise into your hand. Exhale slowly. Take another breath in, and feel your chest rise into your hand. As you exhale, feel your chest relax. Massage upside-down C-strokes over your heart and lungs. As you inhale, imagine a majestic rainbow in your heart.

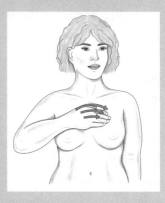

As you exhale, release a cloud from your chest. Repeat ten times.

Step 8

Lightly tap the fingertips of both hands over your sternum at the inter-costal nodes. This percussion can loosen stagnant mucus. Sound therapy has been shown to have healing benefits on the body. Visualize the sound of the thumping vibrating down into your cells. This is where your T cell–maturing thymus is located, above your heart. It stores immature white blood cells and gets them ready to become active T cells to mount an immune response that will help destroy infected and nefarious cells (including cancer). It's also the area where some of your breast fluid drains into the mammary lymph nodes. As you tap your chest, imagine all the benefits of your thymus.

Step 9

Lie down. It's easiest to access your rib cage from a prone position. Lift your right hand over your head if that's comfortable. I recommend placing a pillow under that arm so it can completely relax. Place your other hand on your rib cage, fingers pointing 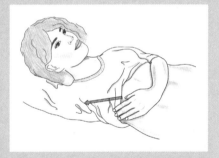 toward your side waist. You will feel the spaces between your ribs. Put your fingers in between as many ribs as you can reach. **Gently** massage C-strokes **inward** and **upward** diagonally toward your armpit. Take deep breaths into your hands, and let the exhale slowly escape through your mouth. Repeat ten times.

Step 10

Massage the fluid from your side waist with overlapping C-strokes **up** to your armpit. Repeat five times.

Step 11

Repeat Steps 3 and 4: Massage the axillary lymph nodes in your armpits again five times.

Step 12

Repeat Steps 9 to 11 on your opposite side.

Step 13

Place both your hands underneath your breasts, your fingers facing each other. You will be able to feel the spaces between your ribs. Delicately pump your hands medially and up toward the center of your chest. This is the second drainage pattern of the lungs. Repeat ten times.

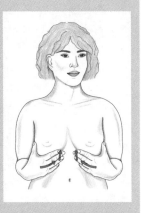

Step 14

Repeat Step 7: Draw rainbows over your chest.

Step 15

Repeat Step 6: Stimulate the intercostal nodes at your sternum.

Step 16

Repeat Step 8: Tap the intercostals at your sternum.

Step 17

Do deep diaphragmatic breathing. This can be done sitting, standing, or lying down. I recommend lying down as it enables you to breathe for a longer time and more comfortably. This exercise is essential to getting more oxygen into the lungs, especially if you're recovering from lung issues. Place one hand on your chest, your other hand on your abdomen.

1. Inhale deeply through your nose, expanding your abdomen into your hands. Exhale through your mouth, and let your stomach soften and recede toward your spine. Inhale again. Use your breath to color in the circumference of your abdomen. Exhale. Feel the posterior (back) of your body and the surface beneath you. This is your solar plexus chakra, between your navel and your sternum.

2. Breathe into the sides of your torso, your side waist. Feel your inhales expand your rib cage on either side.

3. Inhale higher now, bringing the breath all the way into your sternum. Feel the expansion into your heart and breastbone. Allow your breath to lift the front of your body from your stomach to your chest. Exhale slowly and think about letting go of whatever no longer serves you. Repeat three times.

4. Imagine that there's a cotton ball in your abdomen. As you inhale, let that cotton ball rise up past your lungs and into your heart. As you exhale, massage rainbows on your chest with your top hand as you visualize the cotton ball sinking back down to your abdomen. Repeat five times.

5. Inhale all the way up to your shoulders, filling your heart and your lungs with air. Exhale slowly, allowing the back of your body to softly relax into the surface beneath you. Repeat three times.

Step 18
Repeat Step 1: Stimulate the right and left supraclavicular lymphatic nodes at the base of your neck.

ALSO HELPFUL: Eating a diet rich in anti-inflammatory foods (see the list on page 272) and herbs (see page 279), drinking green tea, and incorporating eucalyptus steams and saunas.

Good Sleep

Many of my clients tell me they have trouble sleeping. This is what I tell them: you will improve every function in your body by getting proper sleep. It's that important.

We all know we need a good night's sleep, but how many of us actually get it on a regular basis? Sleep deprivation can be responsible for symptoms such as memory loss, weight gain, irritability, hormone fluctuations, infertility, depression, and respiratory and cardiac disease and can lead to dangerous accidents. Getting a good night's sleep is also essential to your immune health. As you read in chapter 2, the glymphatic vessels in your brain narrow as you age, making it harder for plaque to be properly cleared. With sufficient sleep and lymphatic drainage, you can encourage healthy brain detoxification.

This sequence is structured around the vagus nerve, the largest cranial nerve in the body, which extends from your brain through your face into your thorax and then down into your abdomen. It transmits information to and from the surface of the brain to organs throughout your body and is responsible for regulating internal organ functions such as heart rate, respiratory rate, and even some reflex actions such as coughing and sneezing. It's part of the digestive and nervous system circuit that links the neck, heart, lungs, and abdomen to the brain. In Latin, *vagus* means "wanderer." This is a beautiful image to describe the meandering path the vagus nerve takes through your body. It's also connected to your vocal cords as it runs through the right side of your throat, which is why you'll be humming in this sequence. Singing, humming, or chanting is a wonderful way to engage this nerve.

In addition, the vagus nerve is part of the autonomic nervous system, which controls the parasympathetic rest-and-digest response. Your vagal tone is measured by tracking your heart rate alongside your breathing rate. Your heart rate speeds up on your inhales and slows down when you exhale. The bigger the difference between your inhalation heart rate and your exhalation heart rate, the higher your vagal tone. You want a higher vagal tone; it means that your body can relax more quickly after a stressful situation. It's one of the reasons why breathing is so beneficial during meditation. Increasing the vagal tone of your body is the key to engaging the vagus nerve, which will enable you to move more speedily out of the fight-or-flight sympathetic state and downregulate into the parasympathetic state, which enables heart rate, blood pressure, and digestion to return to homeostasis. As a result, it will be easier for you to fall asleep and stay asleep.

This sequence is designed to assist your body to enter the parasympathetic state and enable you to rest, restore, and properly process all the food and emotions from your daily activities. The free circulation of lymph and removal of toxins and waste in your tissues and digestive tract will not only help you sleep more soundly but will also benefit your immune health.

For this sequence, I recommend you lie down. If you are familiar with yoga, you might assume the suptabadhakonasana (reclining butterfly) or supported savasana (final resting corpse) pose. Basically, lie down with some pillows stacked underneath your back; you want to make sure your head is higher than your heart. You can either bring the soles of your feet together in a butterfly position or stretch your legs straight out in front of you. If that's not comfortable or if you don't have enough pillows, that's fine, too. You can lie down flat with one pillow under your knees and another behind your head. Just get comfy!

Step 1

Stimulate the right and left supraclavicular lymphatic nodes at the base of your neck just above your collarbone. Press your fingertips **down** into the hollows of your collarbone. Make a J motion as you press **lightly down** and **out** toward your shoulders. Repeat ten times.

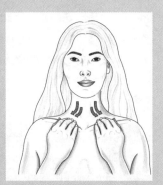

Step 2

Perform the "Neck" sequence. There are three steps:

1. Place both your palms at the base of your neck. Pulse the skin **gently** as you stroke **downward** toward your collarbone. Repeat ten times.
2. Place your hands higher so your pinky fingers rest in the groove behind your ears, your fingertips pointing diagonally toward your ears. Use your palms to stretch the skin **downward** toward your neck. Repeat five times.
3. Make light brushstrokes from behind your ears all the way down your neck. Repeat five times. Swallow once.

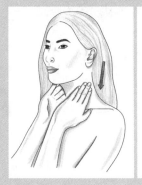
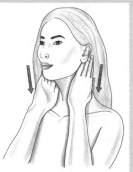
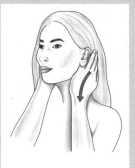

Step 3

Perform the "Spock" sequence: Separate your fingers between your middle and ring fingers (Spock-like). Place your middle and index fingers behind your ears in the cartilage groove and your ring and pinky fingers in front of your ears. **Gently** massage **back** and **downward** in a C-stroke. Repeat ten times. This stimulates both the pre- and retroauricular lymph nodes of your ears. This should be a rhythmic, nurturing movement. Swallow once.

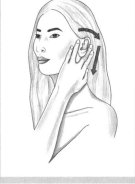

Step 4

Place your hands behind your ears, your pinky fingers resting in the cartilage groove. Massage C-strokes toward the back of your scalp, then **downward** toward your neck. Repeat ten times.

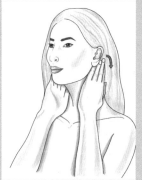

Step 5

Do ear pulls:

1. With your index finger and thumb, *gently* stretch the cartilage inside your earlobe **downward** and **outward**, toward the back of your head. Hold for ten seconds, breathing deeply. Open and close your mouth twice. Release your earlobe and swallow once.

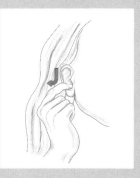

2. Move your index finger and thumb to another spot inside your earlobe. *Gently* stretch the lobes **downward** and **outward**, toward the back of your head. Hold for ten seconds, breathing deeply. Open and close your mouth twice. Release your earlobe and swallow once.

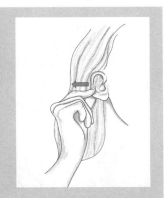

3. Continue working all along your earlobe up to the very top of your ear. **Gently** stretch the cartilage in each place **outward** toward the back of your scalp, and hold for ten seconds. (If you are wearing earrings, be mindful to avoid them.)

4. With your index finger inside your ear, grab the small pointed nodule in front of your ear where it meets your cheek, called the tragus. Pull in toward your cheek. Hold for ten seconds. Move the nodule up and down and back toward your cheek again. Release your ear, open and close your mouth twice, and swallow once.

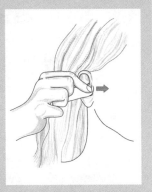

Step 6
Repeat Step 5 on your opposite ear.

Step 7
Repeat Step 3, the "Spock" sequence.

Step 8

Massage behind your ear and down your neck. Swallow twice. Because the vagus nerve is involved with the carotid sinus, these movements will help promote vagal tone.

Step 9

Place your fingertips at the base of your skull, in the occipital ridge. With your fingers touching, **gently** walk your fingertips along the ridge, then glide them **down** your neck, the way a waterfall streams down a mountain. Repeat ten times.

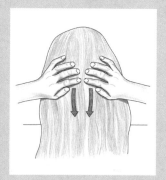

Step 10

Place one hand on your chest. Take a deep breath into your heart. Exhale and say, "Hawwww." Repeat three times. Tap **lightly** on your sternum. Repeat ten times.

Step 11

Draw rainbows over your chest: Place the palm of one hand in the center of your chest, over your breastbone. Take a slow, deep breath, and feel your chest rise into your hand. Exhale slowly. Take another breath in, and feel your chest rise into your hand. As you exhale, feel your chest relax. Massage upside-down C-strokes over your heart and lungs. As you inhale, imagine a majestic rainbow in your heart. As you exhale, release a cloud from your chest. Repeat ten times.

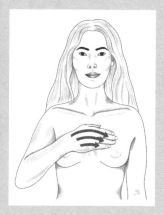

Step 12

Do deep abdominal breathing: With your hands on your abdomen, take a slow, deep breath in. As you inhale, expand your abdomen into your hands. As you exhale, relax. Breathe into the sides of your torso, your side waist. Feel your inhales and exhales reach your rib cage on either side.

As you inhale, bring the breath all the way into your heart. Imagine your favorite flower blossoming with each breath you take. Feel the expansion into your heart and lungs. As you exhale, visualize the stem of the flower at the base of your navel, rooted and strong. Inhale again. Use your breath to color in the entire circumference of your abdomen with a field of flowers. As you slowly exhale, see the wind making the flowers dance.

Repeat three times.

Step 13

With the palm of one hand, make overlapping circles all around your colon: up your right side, across your abdomen, and down your left side. Make circles under your navel toward your left hip. Imagine you are drawing suns and moons all over your abdomen. Visualize 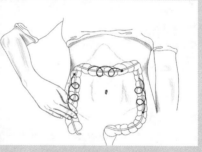 your belly radiant like a clear sky. Allow your strokes to be nourishing and simple. Use as much of your palm and fingers as possible. Feel the surrounding tissue melt underneath your hands. This is the lymphatic way. Circle your abdomen at least ten times.

Step 14

Massage small circles around the circumference of your belly button. You can use a little more pressure here, as this is where your deeper network of lymph resides. If you find any tight areas, spend some time nourishing yourself there.

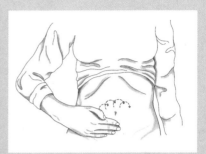

Step 15

Repeat Step 13: Make overlapping circles on your colon, kneading your belly happily like a purring cat. Revisit any areas needing more attention.

Step 16

Breathe from your stomach into your heart, exhaling slowly. Repeat "Hum" three times. SMILE!

Step 17

Repeat Step 1: Stimulate the right and left supraclavicular lymphatic nodes at the base of your neck.

Step 18

Make light brushstrokes on your face from your chin and cheeks to your ears, from your forehead to your ears, and down your neck.

Step 19

Rub your palms together vigorously. Once they heat up, place them over your eyes. Hold them there as you breathe deeply three times and visualize a violet light from the crown of your head to your toes and emanating out from your body. As you release your hands, press your palms into your cheekbones.

   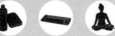

WOMEN'S HEALTH

Breast Care
Premenstrual Syndrome and Perimenopausal/ Menopausal Symptom Relief
Pregnancy and Postpartum

Breast Care

Most women don't touch their breasts regularly, unless they're breastfeeding or as part of lovemaking—though usually it's the lover who is doing the touching. I want you to become intimate with the landscape of your breasts and the 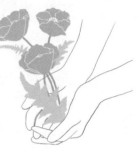 terrain of your breast tissue. You may be used to touching your breasts only when you're doing breast screenings—which can be scary! But I want you to cultivate loving-kindness and recognize that when you are massaging your breasts, you are improving the lymphatic circulation to help clear stagnation in the tissues and create a more harmonious and healthy landscape in your chest. It's common to carry tension in your shoulders and neck, but tension gets trapped throughout the rest of your body, too. Your breasts are associated with your fourth, or heart chakra, which represents your emotions. Think for a moment how easy it is to allow stress to set you out of balance *emotionally*; that change impacts you *physiologically*. Even if you deal with stress mentally, it's a good idea to tend to yourself physically.

Hormonal fluctuations throughout the month can lead to painful symptoms in your breasts, especially tenderness and swelling. Contraception such as birth control pills can cause a temporary increase in your breast

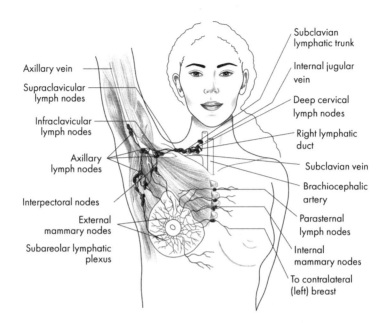

Axillary vein

Supraclavicular
lymph nodes

Infraclavicular
lymph nodes

Axillary
lymph nodes

Interpectoral nodes

External
mammary nodes

Subareolar lymphatic
plexus

Subclavian
lymphatic trunk

Internal jugular
vein

Deep cervical
lymph nodes

Right lymphatic
duct

Subclavian vein

Brachiocephalic
artery

Parasternal
lymph nodes

Internal
mammary nodes

To contralateral
(left) breast

size; lack of exercise can exacerbate lymph stagnation; weight gain can add fat cells to your breasts, increasing your estrogen level and the risk of developing breast cancer; and alcohol consumption, which is also a cancer risk as excessive drinking can alter your cellular DNA, can change the landscape of your breasts as well.

It's challenging to move lymph in your breasts with exercise alone; fortunately, lymphatic self-massage is phenomenal for improving breast congestion and lymph flow. Lymphatic drainage is recommended by doctors and surgeons if you've had breast cancer, a lumpectomy, lymph node removal, surgery, reconstruction, radiation, biopsies, or breast reduction, lifts, or augmentation. The gentle techniques of lymphatic massage are beneficial for healing trauma in the tissues, even if the surgery was an elective breast augmentation. It's also powerful for anyone who is interested in maintaining breast health. If you've had treatment for breast cancer, you will want to work with a Certified Lymphedema Therapist. Please refer to the Lymph-edema sections of this book including the "Arm Sequence for Lymph-edema" and "Breast Sequence for Lymphedema" on pages 240 and 251 to help re-route fluid and manage any inflammation you be experiencing.

Many women have dense breast tissue, no matter what size their breasts may be, which makes it harder to detect cancer in mammograms. For the past twenty years, the majority of my practice has been made up of cancer patients. The percentage of women who are diagnosed with breast cancer is staggering; currently, one out of every four women will develop it. Countless young women have come to me because cancer runs in their family or they have a cancer gene mutation and want to tend to their health in any way they can in the hope of avoiding this disease.

Breast tenderness, breast density, and calcifications aren't something you need to live with forever. You can soften the landscape of your breasts with a gentle, nurturing touch. Some of my clients' mammograms have shown a major reduction in breast density from the previous year thanks to their self-massage routines. Not only is it important to maintain lymph flow in your breasts to reduce toxic buildup, it allows for cancers to be seen more easily in mammography imaging.

If you're breastfeeding, check with your doctor before doing this se-quence. Once you have clearance from your physician that it's okay, this sequence can help support lactation and stave off mastitis and clogged milk ducts. Just use an extra-light touch and do fewer repetitions.

When you use your hands, you will increase your sensitivity and will eventually be able to feel a shift in the quality of your breast tissue. I've had clients tell me that the tenderness in their breasts subsided during their periods, and others have said that this massage helped alleviate puffiness near their armpits that accumulated during menopause. I've also seen scar tissue from surgeries improve.

A lot of women (and men, too) have had self-judgment, fear, and disappointment about how their breasts look and feel—to themselves and to others—at some point in their lives. My hope is for you to cultivate body acceptance. I invite you to create a new relationship with your breasts, one of radical gratitude and grace. Lymphatic self-massage is about looking beneath the outer skin into the nutrient-rich environment where your cells, fluid, and immunity create an amazing ecosystem of health.

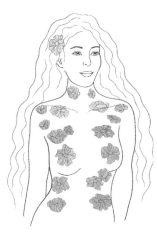

Breast Care Sequence

If you are currently undergoing treatment for breast cancer or have a lump in your breast, please consult your physician before beginning this sequence. If you have lymphedema or are at risk due to cancer treatment, please refer to the "Breast Sequence for Lymphedema" on page 251.

Use skin-on-skin contact as often as possible. It's okay to massage yourself over your clothing, but do get into the habit of massaging directly on your skin for maximum benefit.

Step 1

Stimulate the right and left supraclavicular lymphatic nodes at the base of your neck just above your collarbone. Press your fingertips **down** into the hollows above your collarbone. Make a J motion as you press **lightly down** and **out** toward your shoulders. Repeat ten times.

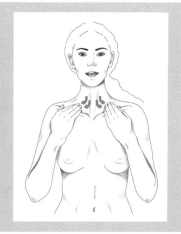

Step 2

Stimulate the axillary lymph nodes in your armpit. There are three steps:

1. Place your hand inside your armpit, your index finger resting **gently** in the groove of your armpit. Pulse **upward** into your armpit. Repeat ten times.
2. Move your hand **down** the side of your torso. This region contains breast tissue, which is essential to drain. With the palm of your hand, make C-strokes **up** the side of your torso into your armpit. Repeat ten times.
3. Lift your arm and place your hand into your armpit. Pump **downward** over your armpit ten times. Release your arm.

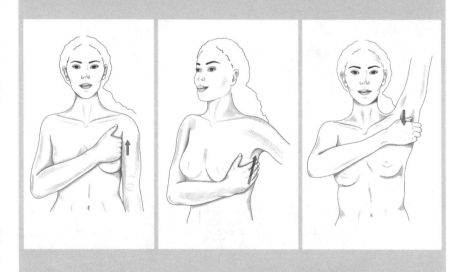

Step 3

Stimulate your shirt-collar lymphatic zone: Place your hands on top of your shoulders, your elbows pointing straight in front of you. Inhale, then drop your elbows as you exhale, keeping your fingertips on your shoulders. Repeat five times. This helps move lymphatic fluid from the back of your neck to the drains above your collarbone.

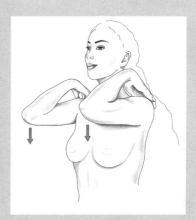

Step 4

Draw rainbows over your chest: Place the palm of one hand in the center of your chest, over your breastbone. Take a slow, deep breath, and feel your chest rise into your hand. Exhale slowly, feeling your chest relax. Take another breath in, and feel your chest rise into your hand. As you exhale, feel your chest relax. Massage upside-down C-strokes over your heart and lungs. As you inhale, imagine a majes-

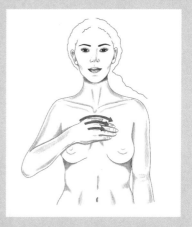

tic rainbow in your heart. As you exhale, release a cloud from your chest. This is where your heart chakra lies; treat it with acceptance, self-love, and tenderness. Repeat ten times.

Step 5

Massage the top of your breast: Place the palm of your hand above your breast, your fingertips facing your armpit. **Gently** massage C-strokes over the top of your breast toward your armpit. Repeat five times.

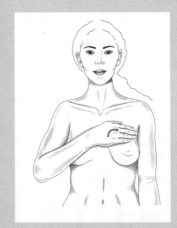

Step 6

Repeat Step 2: Stimulate the axillary lymph nodes in your armpit three times.

Step 7

Massage your breast under the bra line: Place your palm underneath your breast, your fingertips pointing toward the side of your torso. **Gently**, like a wave, massage C-strokes toward the side of your torso. Continue massaging fluid **up** the side of your torso into your armpit. Repeat three times.

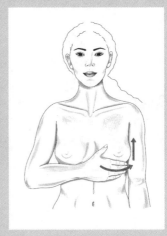

Step 8

Place your hands on your sternum into the grooves of your intercostals. **Very gently**, press **in** and **out**. You are working only on the fluid layer, so resist the urge to press deeply. Inhale and exhale. Some of your breast fluid will drain into the mammary chain of lymph nodes. This move also helps pump air out of your lungs. Repeat ten times.

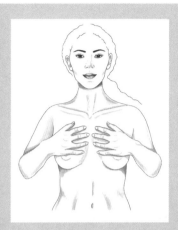

Step 9

Pump your rib cage: These next two steps are easier to access if you are reclining or lying down, although it's not necessary. Place your hand over your rib cage. Your fingers will rest in the grooves between the ribs. As you breathe in, expand the air into your ribs. As you exhale, **gently** massage C-strokes **upward** with your hand into the soft spaces of your ribs. This area gets tender from time to time. Spend a few extra moments cradling your ribs. This is a powerful protective area that shields your vital organs. You want to soften and melt the tension without using force.

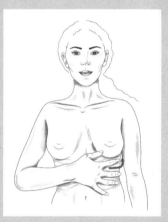

Step 10

With your hand still on your rib cage under your breast, pump your breast tissue **diagonally upward** toward your armpit. This is easiest if you're lying down. Avoid moving fluid into your nipple. Repeat five times.

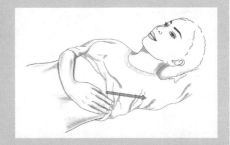

Step 11

Lightly tap your sternum. Visualize the sound of the thumping down into your cells. This is where your T cell–maturing thymus is located, above your heart. The thymus stores immature white blood cells and gets them ready to become active T cells to mount an immune response that will help destroy infected and nefarious cells. As you tap your chest, imagine all the benefits of your thymus.

Step 12

Repeat Step 5: Massage the top of your breast.

Step 13

Gently knead your breast all around the circumference. Feel free to use your whole hand and the pads of your fingertips— whatever feels comfortable. Massage overlapping C-strokes to move fluid away from your nipple. Think of the sun's rays radiating from the nipple **outward**. Some of the fluid in your medial breast will drain into the lymph nodes along your sternum called the inter-

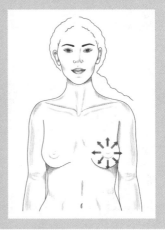

nal chain of mammary lymph nodes, while the fluid in the lateral aspect of your breast will drain into the axillary lymph nodes in your armpit. Do not massage fluid toward your nipple. Spend some time here getting to know your breast tissue. Some breasts are lumpier than others. Some are smaller than others. I want you to get to know yours. Become comfortable with how they feel. You will notice different things at different times of the month. Pay attention to the details and the sensation. If you are feeling tender or if you notice a small cyst, **do not** push on it; focus your thoughts and attention on softening the area surrounding it. Create a soft, nurturing environment here. Don't be shy! I encourage you to take as much time as you need to get comfortable. I often say that the more time you take to get to know your body, the more you are cultivating a new landscape.

NOTE: Make sure to consult your physician anytime you detect an abnormal lump.

Step 14
Repeat Step 9: Pump your rib cage.

Step 15
Repeat Step 7: Massage your breast under the bra line.

Step 16
Repeat Step 5: Massage the top of your breast.

Step 17
Repeat Step 2: Stimulate the axillary lymph nodes in your armpit.

Step 18
Repeat Step 3: Stimulate your shirt-collar lymphatic zone.

Step 19
Repeat Step 1: Stimulate the right and left supraclavicular lymphatic nodes at the base of your neck.

Step 20
Repeat Steps 2 to 17 on your other breast.

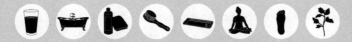

Premenstrual Syndrome and Perimenopausal/Menopausal Symptom Relief

Premenstrual Syndrome (PMS) Symptom Relief

In ancient times, menstruation was celebrated among women and girls as a sacred time of the month. In many cultures it was and still is a welcome time-out to restore—to be nourished and receptive to new energy, in tune with the cycles of the moon.

Now, many women feel inconvenienced by their periods, or suffer pain, cramping, and mood swings. The seat of the sacral, second chakra is associated with sensuality, feelings, intimacy, emotions, and connection. We aren't often taught how to navigate and integrate our emotional bodies. It's commonplace to repress this side of ourselves in our professional lives or mistrust our feelings when they differ from our intellect. This disassociation can build like a wave and apex during ovulation or menstruation.

The pelvic cavity is ripe with lymph nodes that drain the lymphatic fluid of the pelvic region into the lumbar lymph nodes, then to the thoracic duct, where it empties back into the blood circulation. You do not need to work internally to stimulate them. Working externally will increase lymphatic circulation in this area.

- The *external* iliac nodes also receive fluid from the inguinal lymph nodes at the top of the thigh before returning lymph to the common iliac nodes—which is why you'll work your inguinal lymph nodes in this sequence.
- The *internal* iliac nodes receive fluid from the perineum, gluteal region, and pelvic viscera before also draining to the common iliac nodes.
- The *common* lymph nodes also receive fluid from sacral nodes as well as the urinary bladder and parts of the vagina. These lymph nodes then drain into the lumbar lymph nodes, where they meet up with fluid that's been drained there from the ovaries and uterine tubes (and testicles in men).

When I started doing lymphatic massage, one of the most surprising benefits was that it eliminated the pain and bloating I had each month when my period arrived. Virtually all of my female patients check several of the boxes associated with premenstrual syndrome (PMS) on my client intake form. Cramps, breast tenderness, weight gain, moodiness, and other unpleasant symptoms are very common—and can be exacerbated by IUDs, the birth control pill, and other forms of birth control. Many women assume they can't get any relief from painful cramping unless they take painkillers, but many of my clients have found this sequence to be effective. It's wonderful to do when you are experiencing discomfort—whether you are ovulating, menstruating, or at any point in between.

If you've experienced sexual trauma, birth trauma, or any other type of trauma or pain in this area (as a result of surgery or a chronic condition such as endometriosis), your lymph flow can be affected, creating more inflammation in the area. When you do lymph work, you clear stagnant toxins as well as emotions tucked away in the body. Adrenaline accompanies traumatic events, and the significance of that memory is imprinted into the parts of your brain called the amygdala and the hippocampus. The amygdala holds the emotional impact of the event, including the intensity and impulse of emotions. It can also release hormones when the body thinks there's a threat that can have an adverse reaction on the reproductive system. The hippocampus is where episodic memories are stored, moving short-term memories to long-term ones. I've worked with many clients through the last couple decades who have felt a positive shift in how they feel in this area of their bodies once they've cultivated a practice of self-massage.

Menopausal/Perimenopausal Symptom Relief

The onset and symptoms of menopause and perimenopause are unpredictable and vary in every woman. Triggered by a normal decline in the female hormones as women age, symptoms may include spontaneous hot flashes, night sweats, skin changes, thinning hair, weight gain, libido fluctuations, vaginal dryness, brain fog, sleep disruption, mood swings, and depression.

What I discuss with my clients is the deeper issue at the root of these symptoms—the transition in life stages. Menopause ends the "sloughing off" era when the uterus sheds its lining with menstruation. For some, the end of menstruation is a welcome relief. Many women feel more fully able to step into their power at this age—think of the wise elder women archetypes throughout history.

My goal for women is to embrace this time and claim their inner power and self-acceptance. Because breast tenderness, bloating, weight gain, and moodiness don't slough off each month as easily due to menopause, it's common to feel like your breasts are larger and that you have more "side boob" inflammation than you had when you were menstruating. I want you to know you have another innate mechanism at your disposal to flush hormones and excess fluid from your body. Consider your lymph pathways as your means for *flow*. Just because a woman doesn't have her period anymore doesn't mean she doesn't experience symptoms associated with her cycle. It can be challenging to exercise breast tenderness away, and these symptoms can build up in your body over time and cause chronic discomfort. This sequence was developed to help alleviate clogged, fibrotic, or scarred connective tissue and encourage a natural "sloughing off" by accelerating your lymph flow with the power of touch.

When my clients regularly perform lymphatic self-massage, they report experiencing less pain and symptoms during or after their cycle. This sequence is a blend of the "Breast Care Sequence" and the "Abdominal Massage" sequence. I've had so many people write to me telling me that their breast tenderness, pain, and inflammation subsided when they practiced this regularly.

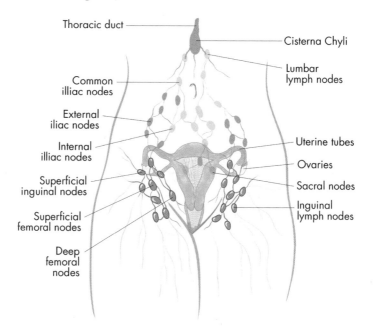

Because the abdomen tends to bloat and fluctuate with hormone changes—some women also get constipated—I encourage you to massage your stomach, too. Once you are adept at this sequence, you can break it into two, alternating between the breast sequence for lymphedema and the abdominal massage.

PMS Relief

Many of my clients say that lymphatic self-massage techniques reduce their dreaded monthly pain symptoms and help to balance out their hormones. (You probably remember that one of the jobs of the lymphatic system is to pick up excess hormones that are too big for the bloodstream to catch.) They've reported less breast pain before their menstrual cycle and find continued relief from chronic pain and PMS symptoms. Generally, I recommend this sequence as needed—usually once or twice a week during ovulation, right before menstruation begins, or if there's pain or cramping with menses. It's a wonderful way to unlock healing and flow in your body.

Step 1

Stimulate the right and left supraclavicular lymphatic nodes at the base of your neck just above your collarbone. Press your fingers **down** into the hollows of your collarbone. Make a J motion as you press **lightly down** and **out** toward your shoulders. Repeat ten times.

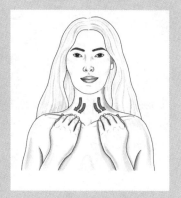

Step 2

Perform the "Neck" sequence. There are three steps:

1. Place both your palms at the base of your neck. Pulse the skin gently as you stroke **downward** toward your collarbone. Repeat ten times.
2. Place your hands higher so your pinky fingers rest in the groove behind your ears, your fingertips pointing diagonally toward your ears. Use your palms to stretch the skin **downward** toward your neck. Repeat five times.
3. Make light brushstrokes from behind your ears all the way down your neck. Repeat five times. Swallow once.

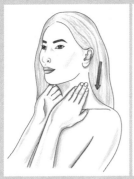 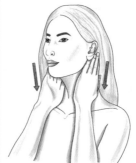 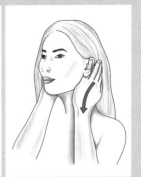

Step 3

Stimulate the axillary lymph nodes in your armpits.

Place your hand inside your armpit, your index finger resting gently in the groove of your armpit. Pulse **upward** into your armpit. Repeat ten times.

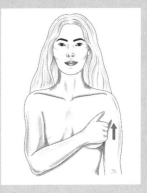

Step 4

Massage the top of your breast: Place the palm of your hand above your breast, your fingertips facing your armpit. **Gently** massage C-strokes over the top of your breast toward your armpit. Repeat five times.

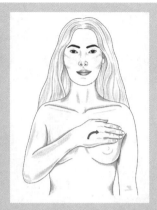

Step 5

Repeat Step 3: Stimulate the axillary lymph nodes in your armpits.

Step 6

Massage your breast under the bra line: Place your opposite palm underneath your breast, your fingertips pointing toward the side of your torso. **Gently**, like a wave, massage C-strokes toward the side of your torso. Continue massaging fluid **up** the side of your torso into your armpit. Repeat three times.

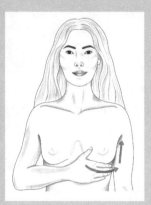

Step 7

Gently knead your breast all around the circumference, moving fluid away from the nipple, radiating outward like the sun's rays. Do not massage fluid toward your nipple. Spend some time here getting to know your breast tissue. Become comfortable with how it feels. You might be used to touching your breast to check for breast lumps, which can be frightening. But your breasts may feel different at

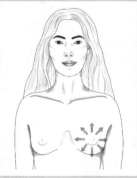

certain times of the month. Pay attention to the details and changes that occur. Infuse your breasts with a loving, nourishing touch. If you are feeling tender or if you notice a small cyst, *do not* push on it; focus your thoughts and attention on softening the area surrounding it. Create a soft, nurturing environment here.

NOTE: Make sure to consult your physician anytime you detect an abnormal lump.

Step 8

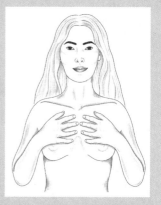

Some of your lymphatic fluid drains to the mammary chain of lymph nodes along the intercostals in your sternum in your torso cavity. Stimulating the nodes at your sternum creates a vacuum effect. Place your hands in the intercostal spaces along your sternum. Feel the indents of your rib cage. **Very gently,** press **in** and **out** along the grooves of your intercostals. Inhale and exhale deeply. This move helps pump air out of your lungs. You don't want to press deeply, as your skin is thin here and you are working only on the fluid layer. This is where your heart chakra lies; treat it with acceptance, self-love, and tenderness. Repeat ten times.

Step 9

Lightly tap your sternum. Visualize the sound of the thumping down into your cells. This is where your T cell–maturing thymus is located, above your heart. The thymus stores immature white blood cells and gets them ready to become active T cells to mount an immune response that will help destroy infected and nefarious cells. As you tap your chest, imagine all the benefits of your thymus.

Step 10

Stimulate your rib cage: Place your hand over your rib cage. This is easiest if you're lying down. Your fingers will rest in the grooves between the ribs. As you breathe in, expand the air into your ribs. As you exhale, **gently** massage C-strokes **upward** into the soft spaces of your ribs. Pump your breast tissue **diagonally upward** 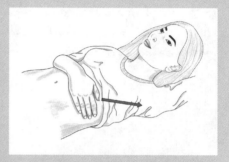 toward your armpit. Avoid moving fluid into your nipple. Repeat ten times. Sometimes this area is tender. Spend a few extra moments cradling your ribs. You want to soften and melt the tension without using any force.

Step 11

Repeat Step 3: Stimulate the axillary lymph nodes in your armpit.

Step 12

Repeat Steps 3–8 and Step 10 on the opposite breast.

Step 13

Place both your hands underneath your breasts, your fingers facing each other. You will be able to feel the spaces between your ribs. **Gently** pump your hands **upward** toward the center of your chest. Repeat ten times. This will also encourage lymph flow to the internal mammary chain of lymph nodes. Repeat ten times.

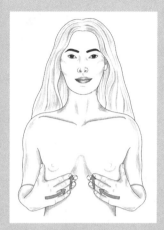

Step 14

Do deep diaphragmatic breathing: Lie down in a comfortable position. Place both hands on your abdomen. Take five deep breaths into your abdomen. Exhale slowly and deliberately. Feel your abdomen rise as you inhale and relax as you exhale. Imagine your thoracic duct bringing all your lymphatic fluid from your pelvis and lower half of your body up the center of your chest and releasing it *clean* and *fresh* back into your bloodstream.

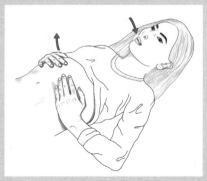
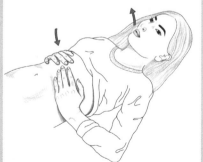

Step 15

Massage your abdomen: Gently massage your abdomen clockwise in overlapping circles. Your colon is shaped like an upside-down C. Follow the lines of elimination; the ascending colon runs from your right hip up to your right ribs. Your transverse colon then crosses 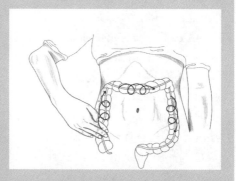 above your navel from the right rib to the left rib. Your descending colon goes from your left rib down toward your left hip, where it meets the rectum. Make small circles all around your colon: up, across, and down. This is your sacral chakra, associated with sensitivity, creativity, intimacy, and self-expression.

Step 16

Make small circles around the outside of your belly button as you breathe deeply. Repeat five times.

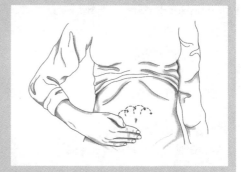

Step 17

Do navel pulls. This is wonderful to help alleviate small
tensions and misalignments
in the abdomen due to movement patterns that put strain
on the muscles and organs.
With the fingertips of one
hand, **gently** pull the edges
of your navel **outward**. Use

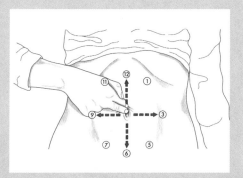

whichever fingertips are most comfortable for you. To begin, pull straight
upward as though your navel is a clock and the time is 12:00 (this point
corresponds to the heart). Stretch and hold the skin for at least one minute in each spot while you breathe in and out. Then move to 3:00 (the
left kidney), 6:00 (the bladder and genital organs), 9:00 (the right kidney), and any other "time" that needs your attention; for instance, 1:00
(stomach and spleen), 5:00 (intestines), 7:00 (intestines), 11:00 (liver and
gallbladder). You may feel a release in other parts of your stomach. I like to
spend a lot of time in this area when I have the time. It's one of my favorite
steps in this sequence; it's very effective in softening the entire abdomen,
as it releases the tension and emotional energy that accumulate when the
connective tissue surrounding the organs gets tight.

Step 18

Repeat Step 15: Massage your abdomen.

Step 19

Scoop from inside your hip bones toward your navel. Begin in front of your
right hip bone. This is where your cecum, ilium, ileocecal valve, and the be-

ginning of your ascending colon are located. It's also the area where your small
intestine merges into your large intestine (colon). This can be tender or tight
if you've had long-standing chronic
constipation. Use the palm of your right
hand to scoop from the front of your
right hip toward your navel. Next, scoop

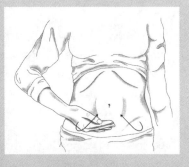

from the front of your left hip bone toward your navel. This is the end of your
descending colon, where your sigmoid colon meets your rectum. This side
can be tender if you've recently been constipated, so be gentle here. You
don't want to stretch the skin—that can be painful! You can create slack in
your skin by pushing toward your hip first, then massaging **down** into your
belly, then toward your navel. Repeat five times on each side.

Step 20

Scoop underneath both sides of your
rib cage toward your navel. Your liver
and gallbladder are located under your
right rib cage, close to where your ascending colon bends to become your
transverse colon. **Gently** create slack
in the skin first, then scoop **downward**
and **outward** from your rib cage toward your navel, similarly to Step 19.

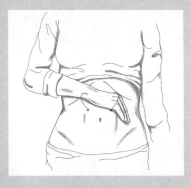

Your stomach and spleen are located under your left rib cage. This is near
the splenic flexure or bend from the transverse colon to the descending
colon. Contour your palm underneath your rib cage and pump **downward**
and **outward** toward your navel. Repeat five times on each side.

Step 21

Repeat Steps 15 and 16: Massage your abdomen and your belly button. Visualize the perfect temperature in your abdomen; the sun is shining, there's a gentle breeze, and the environment is calm and serene. Finish with a few cleansing breaths.

Step 22

Place the palm of one hand above your pubic bone. Take a deep breath into your palm. Visualize a calm lake surrounded by lush trees in your pelvic cavity. Imagine that the sun is setting and there is a brilliant orange glow in the sky. Keep your palm here for a few breaths as you soften all the muscles in this area. Stay here until you feel the ripples of the lake becoming calm and serene.

Step 23

Stimulate your inguinal lymph nodes. Place your hand on top of your inner thigh. Massage C-strokes **upward** to the crease at the top of your thigh. Repeat five times. Repeat on your opposite thigh.

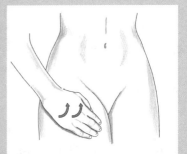

Step 24

Repeat Step 3: Stimulate the axillary lymph nodes of both armpits.

Step 25

Repeat Step 1: Stimulate the right and left supraclavicular lymphatic nodes at the base of your neck.

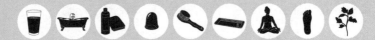

Pregnancy and Postpartum
First Trimester

I don't recommend self-massage in your first trimester. It's a sacred time of the baby's development. As a pre- and postnatal yoga teacher for years, I told my students to use this time to go inward and listen to their developing bodies and changing needs. Even though you may be over the moon at the news of your pregnancy, it's also perfectly normal to have fears and insecurities about how your body feels, hormonal changes, weight gain, or even the acne that may occur at this time.

If you've been doing lymphatic self-massage for a while, once you have clearance from your doctor, you can continue working intuitively while being even more gentle with yourself. Avoid the "Abdominal Massage" sequence when you're pregnant.

Second and Third Trimesters

The following sequences are okay to do at this stage, but do the abdominal massage with a **very gentle** touch. Use **light** brushstrokes over your abdomen. When you rub your belly, use it as a time to connect with your growing baby. I like to tell pregnant women to think of creating space for their child to grow. Your abdominal organs are shifting around, so it's common to get constipated. Gentle massage strokes in the direction of your colon will help your digestion, but again, **be very light!**

These sequences include "Calm Anxiety" (page 148), "Achy Limbs: Arms" (page 215), "Breast Care" (page 189) (simplify, shorten, and go **lightly** so you don't expel any newly forming milk), "Congestion/Sore Throat" (page 82), "Earache" (page 90), "Get Glowing Skin " (page 129), "Headache" (page 99), "Achy Limbs: Legs" (page 223), "Heart and Lung Opener" (page 173), and "Good Sleep" (page 181).

Postpartum

Many women are anxious to feel like themselves again after they've given birth. The best advice I can give you is to have patience and to use this magical time to connect with your baby. The most common question I hear is "When is it safe to do lymphatic drainage postpartum?" The answer is "It depends." Always be sure to get clearance from your physician before you massage yourself. In addition, some of the factors to consider are whether you had a vaginal birth or C-section and whether or not you are breastfeeding. If you've had a C-section, you need to make sure the incisions have fully closed and healed and get permission from your doctor. With breastfeeding, you need to be mindful of developing mastitis, which is an infection in the breast tissue due to inflamed, clogged milk ducts. Breast pain, swelling, heat, redness, fever, and chills are all signs of mastitis that should be treated immediately (often with antibiotics) by your doctor. Never work on yourself when you have an acute infection. If you're breastfeeding, shorten the amount of time you do so you don't detoxify your body too quickly. It's also best to practice self-massage shortly after you've breastfed or pumped. Once you have guidance from your doctor about any other precautions to take, here's a list of recommended sequences you might want to try.

- To promote lymphatic circulation in your breasts, do the "Breast Care Sequence" on page 192.
- If you are constipated, do the "Abdominal Massage" sequence on page 122.
- If you have cellulite, do the "Improve Cellulite" sequence on page 140.
- If you had a C-section or a tummy tuck, do not massage yourself until your incisions have completely closed—which normally takes eight to ten weeks—and after you have permission from your physician. Only then should you perform the "Athletic Injuries, Pre- and Postoperative Recovery, and Scar Tissue" sequence on page 232.

RECOVERY FROM ATHLETIC INJURIES, PRE- AND POSTOPERATIVE RECOVERY, SCAR TISSUE, AND CHRONIC CONDITIONS

Achy Limbs: Arms

Achy Limbs: Legs

Athletic Injuries, Pre- and Postoperative
Recovery, and Scar Tissue

Arm Sequence for Lymphedema

Breast Sequence for Lymphedema

Leg Sequence for Lymphedema

Palliative Care

Achy Limbs: Arms

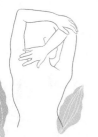

We use our arms every day in nearly everything we do. We tend to take them for granted—only to be reminded of how essential they are once they're injured. Your arms are connected to your heart chakra. We know of their neurological connection because certain sensations in the arms can be health warnings (of an incipient heart attack, stroke, nerve damage, or an inflammatory disease such as diabetes). Our arms also play a role in reaching out: giving and receiving, assisting (working), and nurturing (protecting). We use our arms to create, to give and receive love, to cook, to hold our children. What glory, recognition, and attention they deserve!

It's common to experience swelling in your fingers from time to time. You might notice swelling after eating salty foods, during the hotter months, if you have rheumatoid arthritis, or when you fly or travel to high altitudes. Some of you may have experienced a repetitive strain injury (RSI), such as carpal tunnel syndrome from typing on a keyboard all day or overusing your thumb and fingers scrolling on your phone. Sports injuries such as torn rotator cuffs, tennis elbows, and sprained wrists can also leave stagnant fluid long after the injury has healed. This sequence is a wonderful way to alleviate such stagnation, improve range of motion, and promote lymphatic circulation in your arms, hands, and fingers.

NOTE: If you've had breast cancer, lymph node removal, or radiation, please refer to the "Arm Sequence for Lymphedema" on page 240. Consult your physician first if you are at risk of developing or have lymphedema.

Step 1
Stimulate the right and left supraclavicular lymphatic nodes at the base of your neck just above your collarbone. Press your fingertips **down** into the hollows above your collarbone. Make a J motion as you press **lightly down** and **out** toward your shoulders. Repeat ten times.

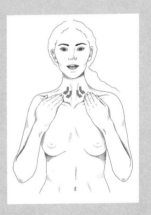

Step 2
Stimulate the axillary lymph nodes in your armpit. There are three steps:

1. Place your hand inside your armpit, your index finger resting **gently** in the groove of your armpit. Pulse **upward** into your armpit. Repeat ten times.
2. Move your hand **down** the side of your torso. This region contains breast tissue, which is essential to drain. With the palm of your hand, make C-strokes **up** the side of your torso into your armpit. Repeat ten times.

3. Lift your arm and place your hand into your armpit. Pump **downward** over your armpit ten times. Release your arm.

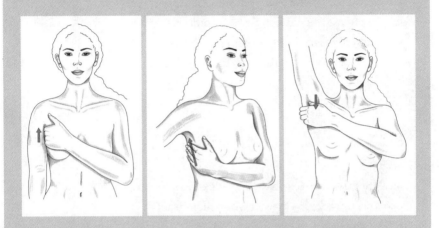

Step 3

Stimulate your shirt-collar lymphatic zone: Place your hands on top of your shoulders, your elbows pointing straight in front of you. Inhale, then drop your elbows as you exhale, keeping your fingertips on your shoulders. Repeat five times. This helps move lymphatic fluid from the back of your neck to the drains above your collarbone.

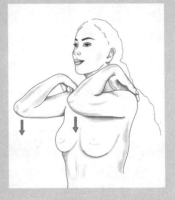

Step 4

Place your hand on top of your shoulder cap. Make C-strokes up and over your shoulder toward your neck. Repeat five times. The drainage pattern here is toward the supraclavicular lymph nodes in your collarbone.

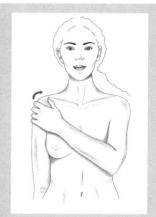

Step 5

Make light brushstrokes on the outside of your upper arm from your elbow to your shoulder cap. Repeat five times.

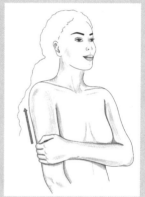

Step 6

Massage overlapping C-strokes along the outside of your upper arm, starting at your elbow and going over your triceps and your deltoid toward your shoulder. Create a wavelike pattern with your strokes. Repeat five times.

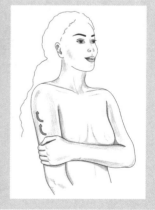

Step 7
Repeat Step 4: Massage your shoulder cap.

Step 8
Make light brushstrokes along the inside of your upper arm from your elbow into your armpit. Repeat five times.

Step 9
Massage overlapping C-strokes along the inside of your upper arm from your elbow crease to your axillary lymph nodes. Repeat five times.

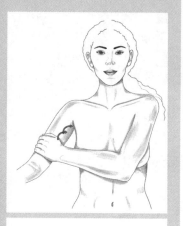

Step 10
Repeat Step 2: Stimulate the axillary lymph nodes in your armpit.

Step 11
Massage your elbow crease, the cubital fossa. Drape your palm over your inner elbow and make stationary C-strokes upward. There are lymph nodes in the elbow crease that receive fluid from your lower arm and hand, so it's important to stimulate this area before you massage your lower arm. Repeat ten times.

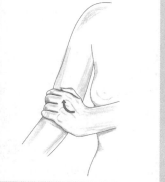

Step 12

Make light brushstrokes from your wrist to your elbow crease. Repeat five times.

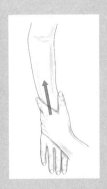

Step 13

Use the pump stroke to massage the top of your forearm from your wrist to your elbow crease. Repeat three times.

Step 14

Massage underneath your forearm from your wrist to your elbow crease. Repeat three times.

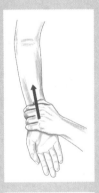

Step 15

Repeat Step 11: With your hand, massage your elbow crease. Repeat five times.

Step 16

Massage C-strokes over the top and bottom of your wrist. With your palm draped over your wrist, massage C-strokes over your wrist. This is a stationary stroke; your hand will remain in one place. If your hand is puffy, you might feel some fluid draining from your hand during this stroke. That's okay; it means you are clearing out stagnation. This area tends to become inflamed due to our constant overuse of phones and computer keyboards, as well as repetitive strain injuries (RSIs). Repeat five times.

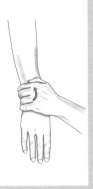

Step 17

Massage C-strokes on your palm toward your wrists. Repeat five times.

Step 18

Raise your arm in the air, over your head if possible. Circle it around clockwise a few times, then counterclockwise. You can start with small circles, then make them bigger and bigger if you feel comfortable.

Step 19

Weave the fingers of your right hand through the fingers of your left hand. Massage the insides of your fingers down to the base. Repeat five times.

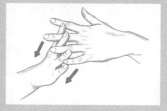

Step 20

Massage each finger separately: Make a cap with the fingers of your hand and massage each finger from the tip of the nail bed down to the finger webbing. Repeat ten times.

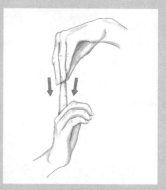

Step 21

Repeat Step 17: Massage your palm.

Step 22

Repeat Step 16: Massage your wrist.

Step 23
Repeat Step 13: Massage your forearm from your wrist to your elbow crease.

Step 24
Repeat Step 11: Massage your elbow crease.

Step 25
Repeat Step 9: Massage overlapping C-strokes along the inside of your upper arm.

Step 26
Repeat Step 2: Stimulate the axillary lymph nodes in your armpit.

Step 27
Repeat Step 3: Stimulate your shirt-collar lymphatic zone.

Step 28
Repeat Step 1: Stimulate the supraclavicular right and left lymphatic nodes in your neck.

Step 29
Repeat Steps 1 to 28 with your other arm, as necessary.

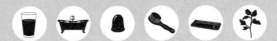

Achy Limbs: Legs

Your legs are your foundation, the roots of your body. They hold you up in the morning and lay you down to rest at night. They provide flexibility throughout the day, carrying out signals sent from your brain and physically grounding you to your feet. Emotionally speaking, legs represent movement, stepping into your role in life, and your ability to flow through things. They can be strong, athletic pillars, but they are also the first of your limbs to become achy and weak when you get the flu. Knee surgery is among the most common surgeries, and hip replacements are run of the mill after a certain age, as is arthritis. These hinges in the body are ripe with lymph nodes to help move out excess inflammation but are also susceptible to lymphatic overwhelm and transport capacity issues because the fluid has to move opposite of gravity, up to your heart. In addition, when trauma and pain build up for years, they can contribute to a plethora of issues in the legs. Studies have found that stress and anxiety can cause tension and constriction in the leg muscles that, over time, can lead to inefficiency and fatigue. By now, you probably understand that when muscles aren't working optimally, lymph movement is negatively impacted. Furthermore, scar tissue from surgeries may have cut through lymphatic pathways, making those areas harder to clear lymphatic fluid from and more susceptible to chronic inflammation.

It's common to experience stagnation in your legs. Most people live a sedentary lifestyle, sitting at their desk all day at their jobs. Or if your work requires you to be on your feet all day, you might find your legs swollen by the end of your shift. Our legs serve as a pump for our circulatory systems. The hinges at your knees and your hips create a mechanism to lubricate your joints and propel lymph. The areas behind your knees (the popliteal fossa) and in your thigh crease are rich in lymph nodes.

Poor diet, lack of exercise, and other genetic factors (such as chronic ankle swelling) can impede lymph flow. If your legs swell at high altitude, due to your job, or when you're on an airplane, it is an indication that your lymph isn't moving well. Remember that lymph flows from the lower half of our body, defying gravity as it moves back up to your heart.

Anytime you do lymph work, you are flushing out toxins as well as emotions that are stored in your body. When you experience a trauma, including sexual trauma, adrenaline rushes through your body and a memory is imprinted into the part of your limbic system called the **amygdala**. The amygdala holds the emotional significance of the event, including the intensity and impulse of the associated emotion. It can also release hormones that are perceived by the body as a threat and have an adverse reaction on the digestive system, reproductive system, and even cell repair over a long period of time.

If you've ever found yourself crying while in pigeon pose on the floor during a yoga class, you know what I'm talking about. Even though you may have mentally processed an event, your emotional body can be retriggered and you may realize that your brain and nervous system have some residual feelings stored in the crevices of your body.

I've noticed that working with lymph nodes in the inguinal area or abdomen can be sensitive for my clients who have been victims of sexual abuse. One of the reasons I teach self-massage is to give you ownership over your body. My hope is that the more you can reclaim those sensitive areas for yourself, the more you can alter the trauma that may be lodged in your sinews and tissues and the more you can harmonize your body and begin healing physically and emotionally.

NOTE: If you have lymphedema in your legs or have had lymph nodes removed from your abdomen or groin or radiation in the lower half of your body, see the "Leg Sequence for Lymphedema" on page 263 for additional must-do steps.

Using Lymphatic Self-Massage to Help Heal Sexual Trauma

One of my virtual clients, Lucy, a young, enthusiastic wellness seeker, was interested in learning about the lymphatic system and how she could incorporate self-massage into her daily self-care routine. She was already dry-brushing her body and jade-rolling her face but had heard so much about lymphatic massage that her curiosity was piqued. During our virtual session, when I was explaining the interconnectedness of lymphatic vessels and how they run through the entire body, including the pelvic cavity and legs, Lucy confided to me that she had experienced sexual trauma when she was younger. She said she'd been in therapy for years but wasn't always comfortable getting a massage because it triggered bad memories. I explained that memories are stored in the body and that one of the benefits of lymphatic self-massage is that it creates more movement in the tissue fluid to rid the body of cellular debris that can accumulate in places that don't get a lot of movement. The other benefit is that when you massage yourself, you are nurturing your body and cultivating a positive relationship with it. I added that at the cellular level, pain and pain relief are caused by two different signaling pathways, but the two pathways aren't necessarily independent of each other. In the brain, neurons in the amygdala that store memory are active during pain and also are associated with negative emotions. When a physical trauma occurs, it registers the unpleasant emotion along with it—which your body will remember. The **hippocampus** is the area of the brain where episodic memories are stored, moving short-term memories to long-term ones. Research shows that when you administer pain relief, you can alter how neurons respond and subdue painful memories in the body. This is one of the reasons I encourage my clients to use meditation and visualization techniques when they work on themselves. It's also why I call the strokes "rainbows" and "crescent moons"—to provide a way for you to signal your amygdala that you are pouring positive energy into your body as you ad-

minister the massage strokes rooted in science and physiology. As I like to say, it's the best of both worlds.

Two months after our session, Lucy wrote to tell me that regular lymphatic self-massage was changing her relationship to her body and helping her heal. I'm so grateful to have had the opportunity to help her.

Step 1

Stimulate the right and left supraclavicular lymphatic nodes at the base of your neck just above your collarbone. Press your fingertips **down** into the hollows above your collarbone. Make a J motion as you press **lightly down** and **out** toward your shoulders. Repeat ten times.

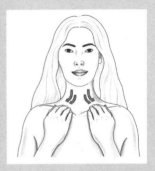

Step 2

Place your left hand inside your armpit, your index finger resting **gently** in the groove of your armpit. Pulse **upward** into your armpit. Repeat ten times.

Step 3

Stimulate your inguinal lymph nodes. There are two steps:

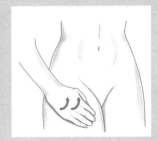

1. Place your hand on top of your inner thigh. Massage C-strokes **upward** to the crease at the top of your thigh. Repeat ten times. Repeat on your opposite thigh.

2. Place your hand on top of your outer thigh. Massage C-strokes **upward** to the crease at the top of your thigh. Repeat ten times. Repeat on your other thigh.

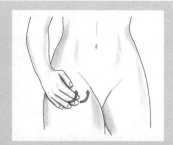

Step 4
Lift each leg six times. This movement stimulates your inguinal lymph nodes.

Step 5
Do abdominal breathing: Begin this sequence with a few deep breaths to create a vacuum suction effect for your lower limbs. Place your hands on your abdomen. Take a deep breath into your abdomen. As you inhale, expand your abdomen into your hands like a balloon. As you exhale, let your abdomen relax. Repeat ten times.

Step 6
Once you have "cleared the drain," you can work on your legs, knees (over your kneecap and behind), lower legs, ankles, and feet. If you'd like to use a little lotion or oil, that's fine.

Massage your upper thigh. You can use one or both hands. There are four steps:

1. Inner thigh: Massage overlapping C-strokes from the inside of your knee **upward** to the top of your inner thigh. Repeat five times.

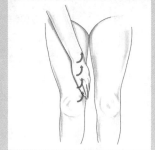

2. **Outer thigh:** Massage overlapping C-strokes from the outside of your knee **upward** toward the inguinal lymph nodes along the outer side of your thigh. Repeat five times.

3. **Center thigh:** Massage overlapping C-strokes from the center of your knee **up** the middle of your leg to your inguinal lymph nodes. Repeat five times.

4. **Back of the thigh:** Bend your leg so you can reach underneath your thigh. With both hands, sweep the fluid from your hamstrings to the front of your leg into your inguinal lymph nodes. Repeat ten times. Pump your inguinal lymph nodes again three times.

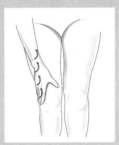 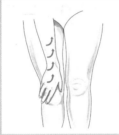 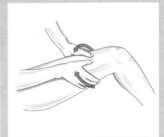

Step 7

Massage your knee. There are three steps:

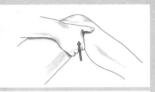

1. Place your hand under your knee. Pump directly into the lymph nodes into the back of your knee (the popliteal fossa). Repeat ten times.

2. Place both hands on each side of your kneecap. Grab the skin on both sides of your knee, and massage C-strokes **upward**. Repeat ten times.

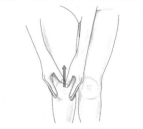

3. Place your hand on top of your kneecap. Stroke your skin **upward** and over your knee. Repeat ten times.

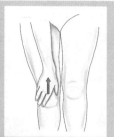

Step 8
Massage your lower leg. There are four steps:

1. Outside of the lower leg: Using both hands, massage the outside of your leg from your ankle to your knee using the pump stroke and overlapping C-strokes. Repeat five times.
2. Inside of the lower leg: Using both hands, massage the inside of your leg from your ankle to your knee using the pump stroke and overlapping C-strokes. Repeat five times.
3. Middle of the lower leg: Using both hands, massage the center of your leg from your ankle to your knee using the pump stroke and overlapping C-strokes. Repeat five times.

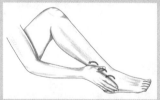
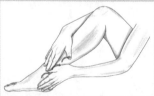

4. Back of the lower leg: Using both hands, massage your calf up into the back of your knee. Pump the back of your kneecap to stimulate the popliteal fossa lymph nodes. Repeat five times.

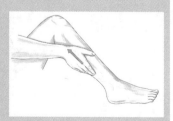

Step 9

Massage around your ankle bones. This area gets congested easily, so feel free to spend extra time here to move out any excess fluid. There are three steps:

1. Place both hands on the outside of your ankle. Massage overlapping C-strokes **upward**. Repeat five times.

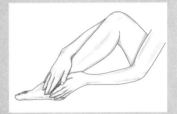

2. Place both hands on the inside of your ankle. Massage overlapping C-strokes **upward**. Repeat five times.

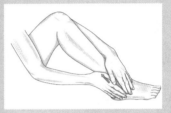

3. Place one hand on the inside and one hand on the outside of your ankle. Simultaneously massage both sides **upward**. Repeat five times.

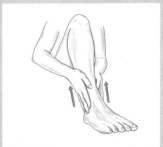

Step 10

Massage your foot: Place your palm on top of your foot. Massage C-strokes **upward** toward your ankle bones. Repeat ten times.

Step 11

Press the pads of the fingertips into the groove on top of your foot between your big toe and second toe. This is a good reflexology point for lymph. Press down onto the grooves between all five of your toes. Repeat five times.

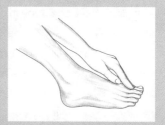

Step 12

Repeat Step 10: Massage your foot.

Step 13

Place one hand under your foot in the pad at the base of your toes and your other hand on the top of your foot. Massage with both hands simultaneously twenty times.

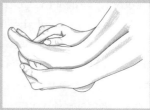

Step 14

Repeat Steps 6 to 10 in reverse order: Massage your leg from your foot up your leg and into the inguinal lymph nodes.

Step 15

Repeat Step 3: Stimulate your inguinal lymph nodes.

Step 16

Repeat Step 1: Stimulate the right and left supraclavicular lymphatic nodes at the base of your neck.

Step 17

Repeat Steps 1 to 15 on your opposite leg.

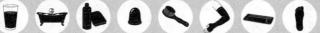

Athletic Injuries, Pre- and Postoperative Recovery, and Scar Tissue

All injuries have one thing in common: inflammation. If you've ever sprained your ankle or broken a bone, you've seen the swelling that naturally occurs as part of the healing process. If you've had surgery to remove your lymph nodes or for other reasons, however, it's possible that your lymphatic vessels have been impaired or cut through. Swelling, pain, numbness, and sensitivity can often linger beyond the period of time you'd expect.

Athletic Injuries, Muscle Soreness, and Recovery

For decades, professional athletes have been getting massages after workouts, big games, and sports injuries as part of the healing process. Doctors, physical therapists, and athletic trainers recommend lymphatic drainage to accelerate healing time as well.

A German study looked at the effect of manual lymphatic drainage on the serum levels of muscle enzymes (the proteins that help cells perform necessary functions) after treadmill exercise and found that muscle enzymes decreased more rapidly after lymphatic drainage massage. They also measured the recovery time after lymph massages as compared to Swedish massage. The results showed that patients who received lymphatic massage recovered faster and had less inflammation than those who had Swedish massage.

We all know the value of exercise and movement for optimum health, but most people who work out regularly will almost certainly experience an injury at some point in their lives. This can have a ripple effect on the body's compensation pattern, in which stronger muscles take over for weaker ones; the biceps in front of the upper arm, for example, which are far more developed than the triceps in the back. A hard workout can also lead to a buildup of lactic acid in your muscles, but lymphatic self-massage will help flush it out of your tissues. Inflammation can also occur after a strenuous workout.

If you have an injury that requires you to take a break from working out, it can take a mental toll, especially if you're used to the positive emotional and physical effects exercise provides. A change in your routine can also be challenging as it lowers the stress hormone cortisol level. In addition, since the lymphatic system is propelled by muscle contractions, a loss of muscle movement can lead to lymph stagnation.

Once you've been cleared by your physician, you can use lymphatic self-massage to promote your recovery. Inflammation can persist long after an injury is healed, and scar tissue can impede recovery as well. If you're able to work your lymphatic drains, depending on how you feel and your range of motion, you can help stimulate new cell growth and get yourself back on your feet faster. Self-massage will also help flush out stress hormones, which will enhance your mood.

Once your acute pain has subsided, follow the sequence related to the area of your injury. For instance, if you sprained your ankle, refer to the "Achy Limbs: Legs" sequence on page 223; if you injured your wrist, refer to the "Achy Limbs: Arms" sequence on page 215, and so on.

Pre- and Postoperative Recovery

Undergoing surgery is among the top reasons to do lymphatic drainage. Pre- and post-op self-massage is wonderfully therapeutic for your nervous system and to increase the circulation of immune cells throughout your body to speed up recovery while protecting you from infections.

Surgeons often need to cut through the intricate network of lymphatic vessels during their procedures. It doesn't matter if your surgery is elective (such as a face-lift, liposuction, tummy tuck, or rhinoplasty) or necessary (such as a knee or hip replacement, cesarean section, or removal of cancerous tissue or lymph nodes), it will have an impact on the superficial lymphatic system.

If you've ever had surgery, you know that healing takes time. Inflammation occurs postoperatively, along with bruising and pain. Some doctors prescribe lymphatic drainage sessions pre- and post-op to accelerate the healing process. When you work on yourself prior to surgery, you will stimulate lymphatic circulation. This can help with scar tissue and keloid (fibrotic tissue) formation. After surgery, you will want to wait until you've received clearance from your physician that your incision has fully closed and healed before doing any type of self-massage in the affected area. Do not massage the site of the operation while your stitches are fresh. Once you have healed and you have your doctor's permission, you can choose the sequence in this chapter that is best suited to your needs. For example, if you had surgery on your breast, refer to "Breast Sequence for Lymphedema" (page 251). If you had a tummy tuck, do the "Abdominal Massage" sequence (page 122). If you had a hip replacement, do the "Achy Limbs: Legs" sequence (page 223). If you've had surgery on your face, any of the following sequences will benefit you: "Earache" (page 90), "Get Glowing Skin" (page 129), "Headache" (page 99), and "Congestion/Sore Throat" (page 82).

NOTE: If you've had lymph nodes removed, lumpectomies, or radiation or are at risk of developing lymphedema, please consult a Certified Lymphedema Therapist. This sequence should be reviewed by your doctor or therapist before you begin a self-care practice. You can find a therapist referral guide in the Resources.

Scar Tissue

Someone once told me to write a letter to a person in my life with whom I no longer wanted contact and then burn it, as that would prevent me from giving away my energy or power to that person. So I wrote a letter and burned it—but I ended up in the hospital with a third-degree burn on my finger. (If you're looking to create such a boundary, I recommend instead that you simply write the name on a piece of paper, fold it up into a neat little square, and place it in your freezer. This will metaphorically freeze that person out of your energetic field and is much safer!) I was left with a very deep scar with ragged keloid edges on my finger. Since I work with scar tissue in my practice daily, I set to work on myself three times a day for months. The results were astounding. I don't have scar tissue buildup, and I don't even remember I have that scar.

Wound care and scar tissue mobilization are practiced by most Certified Lymphedema Therapists because scars from surgery inhibit lymph flow. I've worked on thousands of scars in my practice and constantly teach my clients how to address this issue themselves. But I've also observed in my clients that often, two kinds of scars are bound up with each other: emotional and physical. Physical trauma often results in mental and emotional trauma, which your nervous system struggles to process. So many of the events that create these deep scars—illness, surgery, accidents—affect us physiologically in both mind and body. Unprocessed mental and emotional trauma gets trapped in your tissues, too. As you do the physical work to release painful scars, it is likely that strong emotions will arise; I encourage you to find the support you need to help heal those scars as well.

Physically, scars can prevent lymph flow and range of motion. They can even wrap themselves around organs. This sequence will break up insidious scar tissue. It will soften the fibrotic tissue and reduce keloids (lumpy, raised overgrowths of scar tissue caused by excess proteins in the skin) around your scar. It will also signal your body to reroute lymphatic pathways and increase lymphatic circulation.

Before you massage a scar, make sure the wound is completely healed and there are no openings. Most doctors recommend eight weeks for a wound to fully close, but make sure you get the go-ahead from your physician before you begin a self-massage sequence.

Step 1

Locate the lymph nodes that will receive the fluid from the region where your scar is located. For instance, if your scar is on your foot, the inguinal lymph nodes at the top of your thigh and the popliteal nodes behind your knee are the main drains to stimulate. If you've had surgery on your hand, you will want to stimulate the lymph nodes in your elbow crease and the axillary lymph nodes in your armpit. If you are treating a scar resulting from breast surgery, as the sequence on the opposite page depicts, I would suggest you also refer to "Breast Sequence for Lymphedema" on page 251 (a map of lymphotomes is on page 7).

Step 2

Gently massage the area around, above, and below your scar toward the lymph node clusters.

Step 3

Massage the scar itself. This technique uses slightly more pressure than other lymphatic self-massage sequences do. It's okay to use a little oil if you like. Depending on how long you've had the scar, you might feel some hard, fibrotic tissue underneath the surface of your skin. Over time, you can alleviate the scar tissue buildup by massaging it. There are five steps:

1. Above the incision: With your fingertips, massage a zigzag pattern above the scar toward the ends of the incision. Repeat using overlapping C-strokes.
2. Below the incision: With your fingertips, massage a zigzag pattern below the scar toward the ends of the incision. Repeat using overlapping C-strokes.
3. Directly over the incision: With your fingertips, massage a cross-fiber pattern directly on top of the scar toward the ends of the incision.
4. Massage both ends of the incision. Excess fluid and fibrotic tissue tend to accumulate here.
5. Repeat Step 3: Massage directly over the incision.

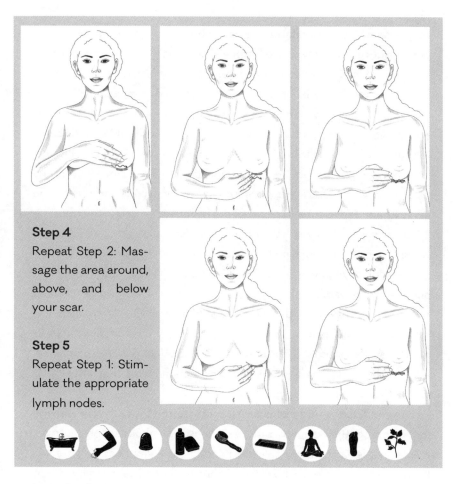

Step 4
Repeat Step 2: Massage the area around, above, and below your scar.

Step 5
Repeat Step 1: Stimulate the appropriate lymph nodes.

Lymphedema

When I was working as a lymphedema therapist at UCLA Medical Center, I recognized the true power of lymph. Lymphedema is a condition in which an accumulation of lymphatic fluid becomes built up in your tissues, causing chronic swelling. It's the result of a blockage in the lymphatic system and is typically located in the limbs but may also affect the torso, head, and other parts of the body. Lymphedema can be the result of genetics (primary lymphedema is a congenital condition in which a person is born with an un-derdeveloped or misdeveloped lymphatic system); trauma to an area of the body; or a side effect of cancer treatment during which lymph nodes have been removed by radiation or surgery (secondary lymphedema). Other conditions that can cause lymphedema include lipedema and lymphatic fil-ariasis. Lipedema is genetic, caused by irregular deposits of fat in the body; because the fat deposits tend to be concentrated in certain areas, they can end up blocking lymphatic vessels. Lymphatic filariasis is a mosquito-borne parasitic disease found in tropical countries in which roundworms enter the bloodstream and eventually obstruct the lymphatic vessels in the limbs.

According to the Lymphatic Education & Research Network (LE&RN), when no more than four lymph nodes are removed during surgery, the risk of developing lymphedema is about 6 percent; if more than four lymph nodes are removed, the risk rises to 15 to 25 percent. At least 30 percent of cancer patients currently have lymphedema, and 10 million Americans suffer from lymphedema. Although a less deadly disease, that figure is more than Parkinson's, Alzheimer's, ALS, and AIDS patients **combined**. Around the world, the figure is shocking: lymphedema may affect 140 million to 250 million people.

Early on, I discovered that when patients started their sessions with me at the onset of their diagnosis and were consistent about lymphatic treat-ments and using compression when needed, their lymphedema often re-mained mild, regardless of how many lymph nodes had been removed. Not only did their risk of developing serious lymphedema diminish, so did their side effects; they experienced less numbness, neuropathy, bloating, indi-gestion, and limited range of motion. In fact, the medical community now recommends early treatment to minimize the proliferation of the disease.

I encourage all of my clients facing lymphedema to take a good look at their stress levels as well. Over time, some have transitioned out of jobs or toxic relationships or simply addressed the feelings and resentments they harbored. I also urge them to establish good health habits, including diet, sleep, and exercise routines. Many of them need some additional support, such as compression bandaging, garments, or pumps, to continue their regime at home. This multidimensional approach helps restore their energy and gives them hope.

The treatment for lymphedema is called Complete Decongestive Therapy (CDT) and is frequently administered in hospitals and rehabilitation clinics by trained Certified Lymphedema Therapists (CLTs). One of the most effective ways therapists can ensure a client's reduction of lymphatic inflammation is maintained is by teaching self-care (manual lymphatic drainage, as well as the pillars you will read about in chapter 5, including diet, compression, exercise, and skin and nail care). It cannot be overemphasized that becoming self-sufficient will yield the best results.

NOTE: If you have lymphedema or are at risk of developing it, please consult a Certified Lymphedema Therapist. This sequence should be reviewed by your doctor or therapist before you begin a self-care practice. You can find a therapist referral guide in the Resources.

Blood Pressure Cuffs and Lymphedema

If you've had breast cancer treatment, you may have been told to avoid having your blood pressure taken or IV needles inserted in the arm on the same side as your cancer. That's because blood pressure cuffs can act like tourniquets—or high-pressure focal compression—and may cause constriction of an at-risk limb if not properly used. Similarly, you want to avoid too many needles repeatedly puncturing your skin during a blood draw because this can increase tissue edema and potentially leave an open wound for bacteria to enter. Because lymphedema is a progressive condition, use an uninvolved or not-at-risk extremity whenever possible if your blood pressure or blood samples must be taken.

Arm Sequence for Lymphedema

This sequence (as well as the "Breast Sequence for Lymphedema" that follows) is designed for those who are at risk of lymphedema due to breast cancer treatment as well as those who have already been diagnosed with it. It's common to experience swelling in the arm to varying degrees immediately after surgery or even years afterward. If you or someone you know is at risk, please find a Certified Lymphedema Therapist to work with.

Some people experience numbness in their arms in addition to inflammation if axillary lymph nodes have been surgically removed in the armpit or as a result of radiation damage. The sooner you begin lymphatic self-massage, the easier it will be to manage lymphedema, should it develop. Don't wait until you see swelling to begin this sequence. **The lymphatic system can swell by one hundred times before it's visible to the eye.** In my career I've seen people who've had forty lymph nodes removed under the armpit maintain a reasonable limb size with constant attention, compression, and self-massage.

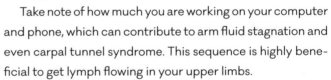

Take note of how much you are working on your computer and phone, which can contribute to arm fluid stagnation and even carpal tunnel syndrome. This sequence is highly beneficial to get lymph flowing in your upper limbs.

If you are at risk of developing lymphedema, you will want to reroute lymphatic fluid to an additional set of lymph nodes. This sequence is similar to the "Achy Limbs: Arms" sequence on page 215. The extra step in this sequence includes stimulating the anastomoses—the pathways of vessels waiting to collect excess fluid that may be stagnant.

There are two anastomoses. The first is the **axillary-axillary anastomosis**, which runs across the chest to the opposite armpit to your other set of axillary lymph nodes.

The second is the **axillary-inguinal anastomosis**, which runs from the armpit down your side to the inguinal lymph nodes at the top of your thigh.

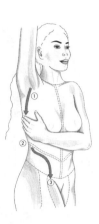

NOTE: There is another anastomosis across your back that connects the axillary node drainage the same way the ones in the chest do. It's nearly impossible to stimulate by yourself. If you want to try, you can place a cloth over a dry brush and **gently** glide the brush across the skin of your upper back from armpit to armpit.

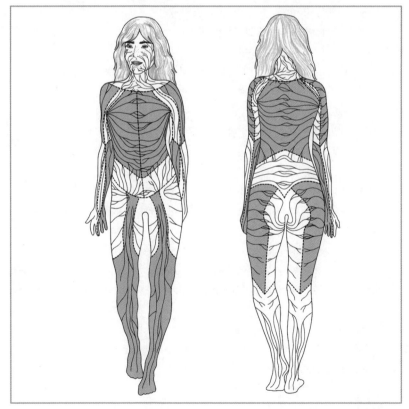

Step 1

Stimulate the right and left supraclavicular lymphatic nodes at the base of your neck just above your collarbone. Press your fingers **down** into the hollows of your collarbone. Make a **J** motion as you press **lightly down** and **out** toward your shoulders. Repeat ten times.

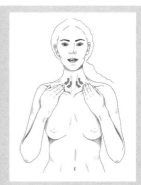

Step 2

Stimulate your shirt-collar lymphatic zone: Place your hands on top of your shoulders, your elbows pointing straight in front of you. Inhale, then drop your elbows as you exhale, keeping your fingertips on your shoulders. Repeat five times. This helps move lymphatic fluid from the back of your neck to the drains at the base of your neck above your collarbone.

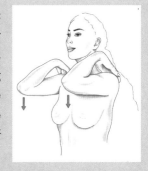

Step 3

Stimulate the axillary lymph nodes in your armpit on the **unaffected** side, the opposite side from the one on which you had cancer or lymphedema; if you had breast cancer on the right side, your left side is your unaffected side. If you had breast cancer in both breasts, you will stimulate both armpits and both inguinal lymph nodes. You will also reroute fluid to both sides of your inguinal lymph nodes at the top of your thighs. There are three steps:

1. Place the palm of your hand inside your **unaffected** armpit, your index finger resting *gently* in the groove of your armpit. Pulse **lightly upward** into the armpit. Repeat ten times.

2. Move your palm **down** the side of your torso. This region contains breast tissue, which is essential to drain. With the palm of your hand, pulse the side breast tissue **upward** into your armpit. Repeat five times.

3. Lift your arm and place your hand into your armpit. Pump **downward** over your armpit five times. Release your arm.

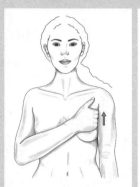 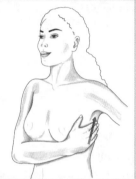 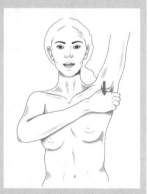

Step 4

Clear the axillary-axillary anastomosis across your chest. Some of your breast fluid drains into the mammary chain of lymph nodes in the middle of your chest, so they will be stimulated in this step also. There are three steps:

1. Place the palm of your hand above your **unaffected** breast, your fingertips facing your unaffected armpit. **Gently** massage C-strokes or rainbows over the top of your breast toward your **unaffected** armpit. Repeat five times.

2. Place your hand on the center of your chest, your fingertips facing your **unaffected** armpit. **Gently** massage rainbows across your chest toward your **unaffected** armpit. Repeat five times.

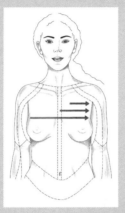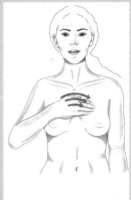

3. Place your hand above your **affected** breast (the side that had cancer), your fingertips facing your **unaffected** armpit. **Gently** massage rainbows across your chest from your **affected** side toward the **unaffected** armpit. Repeat five times.

Step 5
Repeat Step 3: Stimulate the axillary lymph nodes in your **unaffected** armpit.

Step 6
Now stimulate the armpit on the **affected** side, the one on which you had cancer or lymphedema: Place your hand inside your **affected** armpit, your index finger resting **gently** in the groove of your armpit. Pulse **lightly upward** into the axillary lymph nodes. Repeat ten times.

Step 7

Stimulate the inguinal lymph nodes at the top of your thigh on your **affected** side to prepare them to receive fluid from your torso. There are two steps:

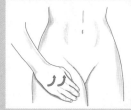

1. Place the hand on your **affected** side on top of your inner thigh. Massage C-strokes **upward** into the crease at the top of your thigh. Repeat ten times.
2. Place your hand on top of your outer thigh. Massage stationary C-strokes **upward** into the crease of your thigh. Repeat ten times.

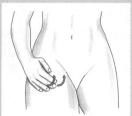

Step 8

Clear the axillary-inguinal, or "Niagara Falls," anastomosis on your **affected** side: **Lightly** brush from your **affected** armpit **down** to your inguinal lymph nodes. Massage from your armpit **down** the side of your torso to your inguinal lymph nodes. There are three steps:

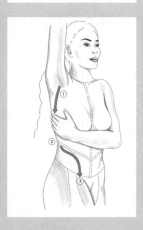

1. Place the palm of your hand directly under your **affected** armpit. Massage C-strokes from your armpit to your waist. Repeat five times.
2. Place your hand on your waist. Massage C-strokes from your waist toward the inguinal lymph nodes at the top of your thigh. Repeat five times.

3. Place your hand on your lower abdomen above your hip bone. Massage C-strokes like a waterfall from your hip to your inguinal lymph nodes at the top of your thigh. Repeat five times.

Now that you've cleared the pathway to the unaffected lymph nodes, you are ready to reroute fluid from your arm by performing the arm sequence on your at-risk limb.

Step 9

Place your hand on top of the shoulder cap on your **affected** side. Massage C-strokes up and over your shoulder toward your neck. Repeat five times. Remember, the drainage pattern is toward the lymph nodes in your collarbone. Do not direct the fluid down your arm; all your strokes are geared toward moving fluid up and out of your arm.

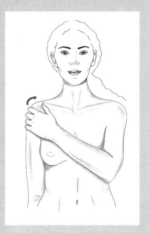

Step 10

With your hand, make brushstrokes on the outside of your upper arm **upward** toward the shoulder cap on your **affected** side. Repeat five times. Then massage overlapping C-strokes along the outside of your upper arm, starting at your elbow and going over your triceps and your deltoid toward your shoulder. Create a wavelike pattern with your strokes. Repeat five times.

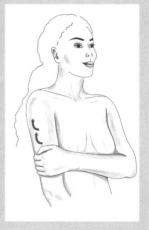

Step 11

Repeat Step 9: Massage C-strokes over the top of your shoulder cap.

Step 12

With your hand, make light brush-strokes **upward** along the inside of the upper arm on your **affected** side. Repeat five times. Then massage over-lapping C-strokes **upward** along your inner arm, starting at your elbow crease and massaging over your biceps to your outer arm and the top of your shoulder. Repeat five times. Pump your armpit five times. Some of the fluid from your arm will naturally go into your armpit because even if some lymph nodes 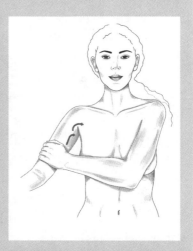 have been removed, lymphatic fluid will still drain into the remaining nodes. In order not to overwhelm the armpit, massage from the inner arm to the outer arm and **upward** toward the collarbone.

Step 13

With your hand, massage the elbow crease, the cubital fossa, on your **affected** side: Drape your palm over your inner elbow and make stationary C-strokes upward. There are lymph nodes in the elbow crease that receive fluid from your lower arm and hand, so it's import-ant to stimulate this area before you massage your lower arm. Repeat ten times.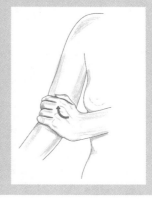

Step 14

Make light brushstrokes from your wrist up the lower forearm on your **affected** side. Repeat five times. Then massage overlapping C-strokes up your outer and inner forearm. Drape your hand at your wrist so it contours your skin. You might feel a swath of fluid under your skin. Remember, less is more. Be gentle. Stop at the elbow crease. Repeat five times.

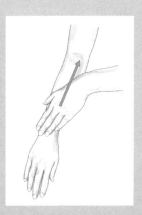

Step 15

Repeat Step 13: Massage your elbow crease. Repeat five times.

Step 16

Drape your palm over the wrist on your **affected** side and massage C-strokes over the top and bottom of your wrist. This is a stationary stroke; your hand will remain in one place. If your hand is puffy, you might feel some fluid draining from your hand during this stroke. That's okay; it means you are clearing out stagnation. This area tends to become inflamed due to our constant overuse of phones and computer keyboards, as well as repetitive strain injuries (RSIs). Repeat five times.

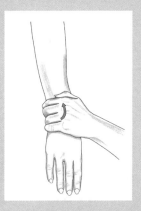

Step 17

Massage C-strokes on the palm on your **affected** side, moving toward your wrists. Repeat five times.

Step 18

Raise the arm on your **affected** side in the air, over your head if possible. Circle it around clockwise a few times, then counterclockwise. You can start with small circles, then get bigger and bigger if you feel comfortable.

Step 19

Weave the fingers of your hands together. Starting at your fingertips, massage the sides of your fingers by moving your hands back and forth as you go, down to the finger webbing. Repeat five times.

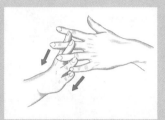

Step 20

Massage each finger separately: Make a cap with the fingers of the hand on your **unaffected** side and massage each finger of the hand on your **affected** side from the tip of the nail down to the finger webbing. Repeat ten times.

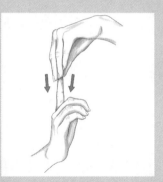

Step 21

Repeat Step 17: Massage C-strokes on your palm.

Step 22

Repeat Step 16: Massage your wrist.

Step 23

Repeat Step 14: Massage up your forearm.

Step 24
Repeat Step 13: Massage your elbow crease.

Step 25
Repeat Step 12: Massage your upper arm.

Step 26
Repeat Step 6: Stimulate the axillary lymph nodes in your **affected** armpit.

Step 27
Repeat Step 8: Clear the axillary-inguinal anastomosis.

Step 28
Repeat Step 4: Clear the axillary-axillary anastomosis across your chest.

Step 29
Repeat Step 1: Stimulate the right and left supraclavicular lymphatic nodes at the base of your neck.

Step 30
Do deep diaphragmatic breathing: Take any comfortable position. Place both hands on your abdomen. Take ten deep breaths into your abdomen, expanding your abdomen into your hands. Exhale, letting your abdomen relax. This will help pump the fluid that you will be rerouting to your inguinal lymph nodes at the top of your thigh.

NOTE: If you have lymphedema, please consult a Certified Lymphedema Therapist before beginning a new exercise regimen.

Lymphedema Relief with Self-Massage

One of my clients, Sharlene, came to see me after postsurgical radiation treatments for breast cancer. Along with scars under her breast from a lumpectomy, she had incisions in her armpit where several lymph nodes had been removed. The breast on that side was slightly more inflamed than the other one due to treatment, felt congested, and was frequently painful. Her range of motion was also limited. I saw her twice a month for about six months and taught her how to do lymphatic self-massage in between appointments. She usually worked on herself three times a week but admitted that there were times when she would skip the massage because she was too busy with her kids. Each time I saw her I could see a significant difference in the swelling of her breast depending on whether she'd done her self-massage or not. Sharlene could tell the difference, too, and told me how amazed she was at how much better she felt after just a few minutes of self-massage, with less pain and tenderness, and that she'd gained back a greater range of motion in her arm, which had been considered to have a "frozen shoulder" after surgery. She was also happy to report that her entire body felt lighter and her general well-being had improved.

Breast Sequence for Lymphedema

If you've had breast cancer treatment, lymph node removal, or radiation, you're at risk of developing lymphatic swelling and scar tissue in the treated breast. Breast inflammation can occur immediately after surgery (even after a biopsy) or a few years later. When the lymphatic system has been damaged or partially removed, the remaining lymph nodes can become overburdened and unable to remove waste efficiently from your tissues, making you vulnerable to lymphedema. Lymphatic self-massage may also improve your range of motion and soft tissue damage.

NOTE: It's important to reroute fluid from your breast to multiple lymph node regions in your body. I also recommend you try the "Arm Sequence for Lymphedema" on page 240. Lymphatic self-massage on your arm can reduce inflammation there.

By now you know that the axillary lymph nodes in your armpit receive lymphatic fluid from the front and back of your torso as well as from your breast tissue. Some of the fluid in your breasts also drains into the mammary lymph nodes along your sternum. If you are at risk of developing lymphedema, you will want to add another step and reroute lymphatic fluid to lymph nodes in the armpit on the side where you didn't have cancer, as well as to the inguinal lymph nodes on the side where you had cancer. If you had cancer in both breasts, you will reroute fluid from your armpits down your torso to the inguinal lymph nodes at the tops of your thighs. We call this the "Niagara Falls" anastomosis. When you reroute lymphatic fluid to other sets of lymph nodes, you are less likely to overburden your lymphatic system. You can stimulate the anastomosis or open another pathway for accumulated, trapped toxins to drain, much the way that multiple rivers drain into the ocean. As you can see from the lymphotome illustration on page 16, excess fluid that may be stagnant due to lymph node removal or radiation has a myriad of routes to depart by; it just needs to be coaxed along a different course.

Recent imaging work has shown that even if lymph nodes have been removed from the armpit, lymphatic fluid can still drain into the remaining axillary lymph nodes, so it's important to stimulate the nodes under both of your armpits. You have anywhere from fifteen to forty lymph nodes in each armpit, so if you had seven removed, there are still lymph nodes in the area that can receive fluid. There are also pathways to the subdiaphragmatic nodes and liver, which is why deep breathing during this sequence will increase the lymph movement. And if you have scar tissue from a lumpectomy, which can adhere to tissue, causing pain and limited range of motion, I recommend you use the "Athletic Injuries, Pre- and Post-operative Recovery, and Scar Tissue" sequence on page 232. When you practice lymphatic self-massage, you will experience less inflammation, see improvement in your range of motion, and possibly gain more feeling in your arms, torso, and breasts.

NOTE: Whenever possible, especially with this sequence, use skin-on-skin contact. It's okay to massage yourself over your clothing, but it's best to get into the habit of massaging directly on your skin for maximum benefit.

Step 1
Stimulate the right and left supraclavic-ular lymphatic nodes at the base of your neck just above your collarbone: Press your fingertips **down** into the hollows above your collarbone. Make a **J** motion as you press **lightly down** and **out** toward your shoulders. Repeat ten times.

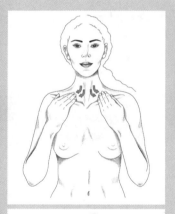

Step 2
Stimulate your shirt-collar lymphatic zone: Place your hands on top of your shoulders, your elbows pointing straight in front of you. Inhale, then drop your el-bows as you exhale, keeping your finger-tips on your shoulders. Repeat five times. This helps move lymphatic fluid from the back of your neck to the drains above your collarbone.

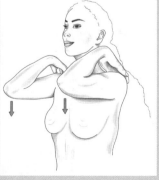

Step 3

Stimulate the axillary lymph nodes in the armpit on your **unaffected** side, the opposite side from the one on which you had cancer or lymphedema. That is, if you had breast cancer on the right side, your left side is your unaffected side. If you had cancer in both breasts, you will stimulate the lymph nodes in both armpits and the inguinals on each side, first on one side, then on the other. You will also reroute fluid to both sides of your inguinal lymph nodes at the top of your thighs. There are three steps:

1. Place the palm of your hand inside your **unaffected** armpit, your index finger resting gently in the groove of your armpit. Pulse **lightly upward** into your armpit. Repeat ten times.
2. Move your hand **down** the side of your torso. This region contains breast tissue, which is essential to drain. With the palm of your hand, pulse the side breast tissue **up** into your armpit. Repeat five times. This clears the side of your torso.
3. Lift your arm and place the palm of your hand into your armpit. Pump **downward** over your armpit five times. Release your arm.

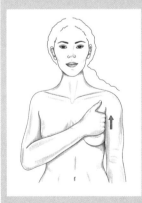 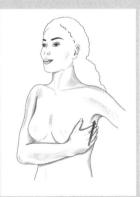 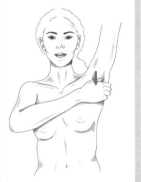

Step 4

Massage your **unaffected** breast first. That is, if you had cancer in your right breast, massage your left breast first or vice versa. It's important to massage both of your breasts to clear as much lymph and inflammation from your chest as possible. This will create the vacuum effect of moving lymph. Place the palm of your other hand above your breast, your fingertips facing your armpit. **Gently** massage C-strokes over the top of your breast, toward your armpit. Repeat five times.

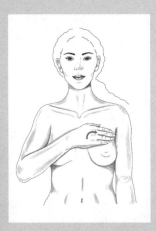

Step 5

Repeat Step 3: Stimulate the axillary lymph nodes in your **unaffected** armpit. Repeat three times.

Step 6

Massage your **unaffected** breast under the bra line: Place the palm of your other hand underneath your breast, your fingertips pointing toward the side of your torso. **Gently**, like a wave, massage C-strokes **up** the side of your torso into your armpit. Repeat three times.

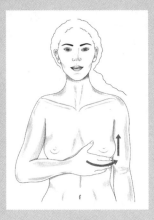

Step 7

Repeat Step 3: Stimulate the axillary lymph nodes in your **unaffected** armpit. Repeat three times.

Step 8

Clear the axillary-axillary anastomosis across your chest. Some of your breast fluid drains into the mammary chain of lymph nodes in the middle of your chest, so they will be stimulated in this step also. There are three steps:

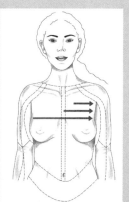

1. Place the palm of your hand above your **unaffected** breast, your fingertips facing your unaffected armpit. **Gently** massage C-strokes over the top of your breast toward your **unaffected** armpit. Repeat five times.
2. Place your hand on the center of your chest, your fingertips facing your **unaffected** armpit. **Gently** massage across your chest toward the **unaffected** armpit. Repeat five times.
3. Place your hand above your **affected** breast, your fingertips facing your **unaffected** armpit. **Gently** massage all the way across your chest from your **affected** side toward the **unaffected** armpit. Repeat five times.

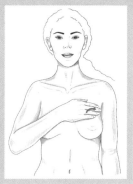
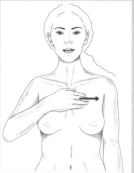
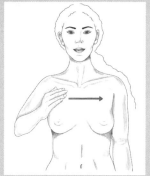

Step 9

Place your fingertips in the intercostal spaces along your sternum. **Very gently**, press **in** and **out** along the grooves of your intercostals. Inhale and exhale deeply. This move helps pump air out of your lungs and stimulates the mammary nodes. You don't want to press deeply, as your skin is thin here and you are working only on the fluid layer. This is where your heart chakra lies; treat it with acceptance, self-love, and tenderness. Repeat ten times.

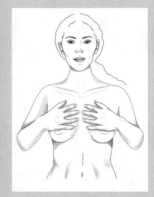

Step 10

Now stimulate the axillary lymph nodes in the armpit on your **affected** side, the one on which you had cancer or lymphedema. If you had lymph nodes removed or radiation, you might still be sore or numb and have some swelling. Please be **extra gentle** and loving. There are three hand positions.

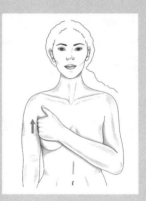

1. Place the palm of your hand inside your **affected** armpit, your index finger resting **gently** in the groove of your armpit. Pulse **lightly upward** into your armpit. Repeat ten times.
2. Move your hand **down** the side of your torso. This region contains breast tissue, which is essential to drain. With the palm of your hand, pulse the side breast tissue

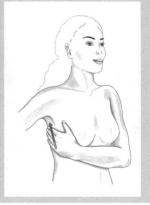

upward into your armpit. Repeat five times. This clears the side of your torso.

3. Lift your arm and place your hand into your armpit. Pump **downward** over your armpit five times. Release your arm.

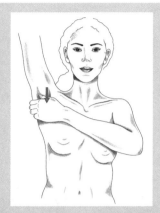

Step 11

Clear the axillary-inguinal, or "Niagara Falls," anastomosis on your **af-fected** side from your **affected** armpit down the torso of your body toward the inguinal nodes at the top of your thigh on the same side. There are three steps:

1. Place the palm of your hand directly under your **affected** armpit. **Lightly** massage C-strokes **down** from your armpit to your waist. Repeat five times.
2. Place your hand on your waist. **Lightly** massage C-strokes from your waist **down** toward your inguinal lymph nodes at the top of your thigh. Repeat five times.
3. Place your hand on your lower abdomen above your hip bone. **Lightly** massage C-strokes like a waterfall from your hip toward the inguinal lymph nodes. Repeat five times.

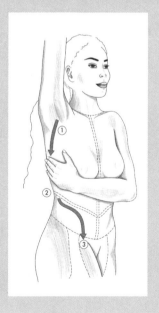

Step 12

Stimulate the inguinal lymph nodes at the top of your thigh on your **affected** side to prepare them to receive fluid from your torso: Place the palm of the same-side hand on the top of your thigh. Massage C-strokes **upward** on your thigh. Repeat ten times.

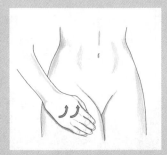

Step 13

Now that you've cleared the pathways (anastomoses), you are ready to massage the breast on your **affected** side, the one on which you had cancer or lymphedema. Place the palm of your hand above your breast, your fingertips facing your armpit. **Gently** massage C-strokes over the top of the breast toward your unaffected armpit. Repeat five times.

Step 14

Massage your **affected** breast under the bra line: Place the palm of your other hand underneath your breast, your fingertips pointing toward the side of your torso. **Gently**, like a wave, massage C-strokes toward the side of your torso. Continue massaging fluid **down** the side of your torso to the inguinal lymph nodes at the top of your thigh. Repeat three times.

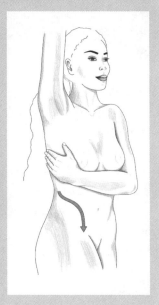

Step 15

Stimulate the axillary lymph nodes in your armpit in your **affected** armpit as in Step 10.

Step 16

Place your same-side hand over your rib cage on your **affected** side, your fingers resting in the grooves between the ribs. As you inhale, expand the air into your ribs. As you exhale, **gently** massage C-strokes with your hands into the soft spaces between your ribs. Sometimes this area is tender. Spend a few extra moments on this step. It's a powerful protective area that shields your vital organs. You want to soften and melt the tension without using any force. This step is most comfortably done in a reclined position. Repeat five times.

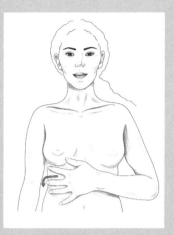

Step 17

Repeat Step 13: Massage over the top of your **affected** breast toward your opposite armpit.

Step 18

With your hand, **gently** knead your **affected** breast all around the circumference, moving fluid away from your nipple, radiating outward like the sun's rays. Some of the fluid from the medial aspect of your breast will drain into the lymph nodes along your sternum, while the fluid from the lateral aspect of your breast is redirected through the anastomoses down to your inguinal lymph nodes. Spend some

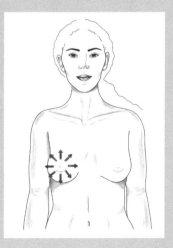

time here getting to know your breast tissue. If you are feeling swollen or tender or if you notice a small cyst, **do not** push on it; focus your thoughts and attention on softening the area surrounding it. Create a soft, nurturing environment here. Imagine a beautiful field of lavender or poppies on a sunny day with a light breeze. You don't want to poke the flowers; instead, relax into the hilly dimension and allow your breast to relax with your delicate, nurturing touch.

NOTE: Make sure to consult your physician anytime you detect an abnormal lump.

Step 19
Repeat Step 13: Massage over the top of your **affected** breast toward the opposite armpit.

Step 20
Repeat Step 14: Massage your **affected** breast under the bra line down to the inguinal nodes at the top of your thigh.

Step 21
Repeat Step 10: Stimulate the axillary lymph nodes in your **affected** armpit. Repeat five times.

Step 22
Lightly tap your sternum at the intercostal nodes. This is where the internal mammary chain of lymph nodes is located, as well as your thymus, which matures T cells that fight cancer. As you tap your chest, imagine your thymus as a blossoming rose.

Step 23

Repeat Step 11: Clear the axillary-inguinal, or "Niagara Falls," anastamosis.

Step 24

Repeat Step 8: Clear the axillary-axillary anastomosis across your chest.

Step 25

Repeat Step 3: Stimulate the axillary lymph nodes in your **unaffected** armpit.

Step 26

Repeat Step 2: Stimulate your shirt-collar lymphatic zone.

Step 27

Repeat Step 1: Stimulate the right and left supraclavicular lymphatic nodes at the base of your neck.

NOTE: If you have lymphedema, please consult a Certified Lymphedema Therapist before beginning a new exercise regimen.

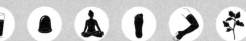

Precautions to Be Taken with Lymphedema, Especially Regarding Heat and Cold

You may have heard that alternating heat and cold therapy is good for the immune system. Although some studies may seem to prove this hypothesis, if you are at risk of developing or have lymphedema, you should proceed with caution. For decades, the lymphatic medical community has advised that you should avoid exposure to extreme temperatures, as they can cause a tissue injury such as a burn or frostbite. One study of gynecologic cancer survivors showed that legs may be more at risk than arms during exposure to heat. I always tell my clients that the rule of thumb about heat or cold therapy is to limit the length of exposure until you know the response of your at-risk body part. If you notice even any slight change, such as swelling, in your at-risk body part, stop immediately—or don't do it at all! There is a risk of tissue damage that will worsen your lymphedema if the exposure to heat or cold is extreme or long enough. Unfortunately, this includes saunas, hot tubs, and topical heat treatments that raise your body temperature.

Leg Sequence for Lymphedema

If you are at risk of developing lymphedema from cancer of the abdominal area, colorectal region, or reproductive organs; have had lymph nodes removed in the abdomen or groin; or have undergone radiation treatments on the lower half of your body, you will want to add another step to the "Achy Limbs: Legs" sequence on page 223. (It's called "rerouting" lymphatic fluid to another set of lymph nodes known as collateral collectors, which I discussed in chapter 1.)

Imagine you're driving on the freeway and your exit is closed or traffic is causing a backup. As inconvenient as this may be, you can just get off at another exit. These detours exist in your body, too: lymphatic fluid can be rerouted to other sets of lymph nodes. This is what we refer to as "stimulating the anastomosis" or opening another pathway for lymphatic fluid to drain.

In addition, if you have leg lymphedema and varicose veins, I recommend you ask your physician if varicose vein treatment is recommended. This condition is often managed by wearing support stockings, and sometimes treating varicose veins can help reduce the lymphatic load of fluid in the tissues and improve lymphedema management.

NOTE: If you have lymphedema, are at risk of developing lymphedema as a result of cancer treatment, or have lipedema or filariasis and experience swelling in your legs to varying degrees, please consult a Certified Lymphedema Therapist. This sequence should be reviewed by your doctor or therapist before you begin a self-care practice. You can find a therapist referral guide in the Resources.

How to Reroute the Two Anastomoses

Inguinal-axillary: Massage from the inguinal lymph nodes at the top of the thigh of your **affected** leg up your hip and the side of your torso into the axillary lymph nodes in the same-side armpit. For example, if your right leg is swollen, massage from your right inguinal lymph nodes up your waist on your right side into your right armpit and stimulate the axillary lymph nodes in that armpit.

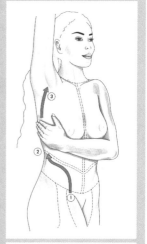

Inguinal-inguinal: Massage from the inguinal lymph nodes on your **affected** side to the inguinal lymph nodes on your **unaffected** side. For instance, if your right leg is swollen, massage from your right thigh crease over your abdomen to your left thigh crease. Then stimulate the inguinal lymph nodes on the **unaffected** side.

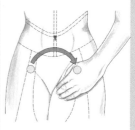

Once you have opened the drains on the **unaffected** side and cleared a path to receive excess fluid, perform the "Achy Limbs: Legs" sequence on page 223.

NOTE: If you have lymphedema, please consult a Certified Lymphedema Therapist before beginning a new exercise regimen.

Palliative Care

Touch during end-of-life care is one of the greatest gifts you can give a loved one—aside from your physical presence and love, of course. I've been called in to work on many people through their last days, and what I've observed is that family members are desperate to help alleviate pain so their family member's transition can be as soothing and comforting as possible. If you're lucky enough to be able to bring in a hospice team, this can be very helpful, as they are usually highly trained in the physical and emotional waves the body goes through as it nears death.

Earlier in this book, I wrote about my mother's death when I was thirteen. I've thought a lot about how I can live with as much freedom in my body and mind as possible so that when it's my time, I will have the tools to let go. I know that no one wants to suffer. Nor do they want to see someone they care for in pain.

Lymphatic massage is a wonderful way to touch someone. It's so gentle and nourishing. It's all about administering a loving touch. Sometimes the person transitioning doesn't want to be touched, so make sure you ask them first. Allow their wishes to be granted.

Hold their hand or feet. If they're on their side, you can **gently** glide your hand over their back. You don't need to follow a protocol or worry about moving lymphatic fluid to certain lymph nodes. Because you have cultivated a self-massage practice, you should be comfortable with a soft touch. Listen to the person. Follow your intuition. Trust that you will know where to place your hand. Even a few minutes' touching can alleviate pain and move energy.

My faith believes that one of the most selfless acts you can do is to attend a funeral. Why is this selfless? Because the person doesn't know you're there. And from what I've seen and experienced, one of the most beautiful acts you can do is to sit at the bedside of someone dying and offer your presence, your love, your friendship, and possibly your touch.

Part III

LYMPHATIC

HOLISTIC

REMEDIES

Chapter 5

SELF-CARE ROUTINES
TO BOOST LYMPH FLOW

There are five pillars of lymphatic good health. In the previous chapters, we've focused on the first pillar, my primary area of expertise, which is lymphatic drainage. But the other four pillars—diet and hydration, skin care and body care, compression, and exercise—are also hugely important to lymphatic health. Attending to each of these pillars will enhance the results of your self-massage practice. When my clients learn that facets of their lifestyle have an impact on where they land on the lymphatic health continuum, they are empowered to make changes so they can maintain optimal results. Whether you're well versed in wellness rituals or you're new to the concept, my hope is that the information in this chapter will help you connect the dots between your physical well-being and your emotional well-being. You'll find remedies that serve as perfect companions to your lymphatic self-care rituals. They will strengthen your immunity, improve your digestion, enhance the appearance of your skin, and help you achieve the "inner flow and outer glow" that's synonymous with good lymphatic health.

PILLAR 1: LYMPHATIC DRAINAGE

Lymphatic massage not only assists your immune system function, but it keeps your body's intrinsic cleansing system running smoothly. By now I hope you've tried a few of the lymphatic self-massage sequences. Doing a simple lymphatic self-massage and some deep breathing a couple times a week will increase lymphatic circulation, which can help reduce inflammation, improve digestion, give you more energy, and move congested toxins out of your body. Continuing to practice this self-care technique will allow you to feel good from the inside out.

PILLAR 2: DIET AND HYDRATION

Making healthy food choices is within your control, but as you know, most of us don't follow a perfectly healthy diet 100 percent of the time. Often we aren't even aware of what harmful chemicals in the form of pesticides and herbicides, antibiotics, or hormones given to cattle end up lurking in our meals.

This is where lymphatic self-care comes in. Choosing what to eat is one of the simplest and most effective choices you can make that will have a long-term impact on reducing chronic inflammation and supporting your body with the cancer-fighting properties of food.

New research suggests that targeted food plans can be helpful in managing lymphatic disorders such as lymphedema and lipedema, as well as any excess body weight that can overwhelm the lymphatic system. These studies show promise for anyone looking to curtail symptoms stemming from lymph stasis. One of these eating plans is the keto diet, in which you eat high amounts of fat, moderate amounts of protein, and very low amounts of carbs so your body will burn fat as its main source of fuel.

This puts your body into a metabolic state called ketosis, which lowers your blood sugar level and turns fat into ketones in the liver; this, in turn, supplies your brain with energy and helps you lose weight. Another eating plan is the Blood Type Diet. Some of my clients have lost weight, lowered their blood pressure, decreased their mucus congestion, lessened their arthritis, and improved their sleep apnea and digestion by following it. The premise is that people with different blood types process food differently, so foods in each food group are categorized as "beneficial," "neutral," or "to avoid" for each blood group.

Further research in the lymphatic medical community has shown that the more you cut back on saturated long-chain fatty acids (found in dairy fat, coconut oil, palm oil, and other vegetable oils such as peanut, canola, and safflower), the better it is for your lymphatic system. This kind of fat can almost double the volume of chyle produced in the intestine, and adding another two liters of fluid to your lymphatic system daily will definitely slow down your lymph transport a lot! Medium-chain and short-chain fatty acids (found in high-fiber foods such as fruits, vegetables, legumes, some nuts, seeds, and whole grains) are processed differently, entering the bloodstream more directly via capillaries in the small intestine. This reduces the amount of extra fluid the lymphatic system needs for optimal functioning.

I point these concepts out because as a lymphatic practitioner, I always tell my clients that in order to maximize their lymphatic health, it's beneficial to find a healthy, sustainable eating plan. Doing so will allow you to maintain the best results with your self-massage routines. You already know that all your body's systems are interconnected, and when you take care of one area, it will have a ripple effect everywhere else.

Foods to Eat

 Start by eating more whole foods and fewer processed foods; more complex carbohydrates in the form of vegetables, beans and legumes, and fruits, and fewer simple carbohydrates in the form of pastries and sweets. You may know this already, but it bears repeating because it's easy to slip back into old patterns of convenience—and before you know it, you're wondering why your stomach feels inflamed and you're waking up congested in the morning. Your lymph flow can be slowed down by what you put into your body!

This list is by no means exhaustive but is a snapshot to show you some of the compounds, especially the anti-inflammatories found in whole foods, that deliver beneficial nutrients and promote microcirculation. Try to add as many of these foods as you can to your regular diet.

- **Raw vegetables and fruits.** They contain enzymes and antioxidants that help your body break down toxins so they can get moved out more efficiently.
- **Purple and red fruits.** All berries (don't forget cranberries, which help promote metabolic function to break down excess fat), beets, cherries, goji berries, plums, cabbage, and watermelon contain powerful antioxidants and vitamins C and K, and most are rich in selenium.
- **Leafy greens.** Dark green vegetables contain the nutrient chlorophyll, which has cleansing properties and beneficial effects on your blood and lymph flow. These include broccoli, kale, spinach, dandelion greens, mustard greens, wheatgrass, and turnip greens.
- **Seaweed.** Sea vegetables contain fiber and wonderful minerals that aid in weight loss and gut health. Seaweed is also rich in vitamins A, B, C, and E, and iron and is a good source of iodine, which helps thyroid function.
- **Pineapple and papaya.** These contain bromelain, a powerful anti-

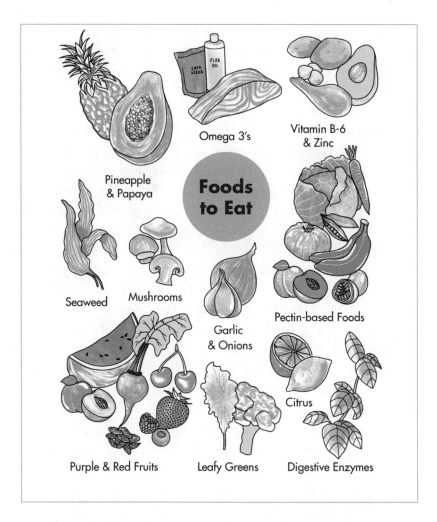

Pineapple & Papaya

Omega 3's

Vitamin B-6 & Zinc

Foods to Eat

Seaweed   Mushrooms

Garlic & Onions

Pectin-based Foods

Purple & Red Fruits

Leafy Greens

Citrus

Digestive Enzymes

inflammatory digestive aid. Many of my clients take a supplement of pineapple or papaya after surgery to help reduce swelling.

- **Citrus fruits.** Oranges, grapefruits, tangerines, lemons, and limes contain enzymes and vitamin C that support your digestion and are good for your liver. In particular, the white pith of a peel contains diosmin, a plant chemical that can increase lymphatic microcirculation and improve the health of your veins. Diosmin is also known as a phlebotonic, a therapeutic agent used to improve blood vessel function.

- **Mushrooms.** These are a powerful antioxidant, as they are rich in selenium, which prevents cellular damage, as well as some B vitamins and vitamin C. They're good for immune support, digestion, healthy cell growth and turnover, and preventing damage to cells and tissues.

- **Foods rich in Vitamin B$_6$.** These help fight inflammation and increase white blood cells and T lymphocytes. You can get this vitamin from bananas, salmon, turkey, tuna, potatoes, chickpeas, avocados, and hazelnuts.

- **Foods rich in omega-3 and omege-6 fatty acids,** such as fatty fish and fish oils (mackerel, salmon, sardines, herring) and seeds (chia, flax), help reduce inflammation and remove fat-soluble waste from your body. They also positively influence the functioning of your immune system's type B white blood cells.

- **Pectin.** This is a type of starch called a polysaccharide, which is found in the cell walls of fruits and vegetables. It has anti-inflammatory properties that nourish the microbiome, repair the lining of the gut, help resolve loose stools, lower "bad" LDL cholesterol, and bind to mercury to help the kidneys process it more quickly. Sources of pectin include citrus fruits, bananas, berries, passion fruit, peaches, and tomatoes, as well as vegetables such as beets, cabbage, carrots, green beans, parsnips, and peas.

- **Garlic and onions.** These contain compounds with powerful medicinal benefits for the blood and immune system. They've been used for centuries for their antibiotic and antiviral properties, making them useful when you have a cold or a virus. Garlic has been shown to be helpful for the heart, blood pressure, cholesterol, and osteoarthritis.

Onions also have antifungal properties and contain cancer-preventing compounds; they're rich in quercetin (a flavonoid antioxidant), an anti-inflammatory that fights free radicals and has been helpful in treating symptoms of COVID patients. Even though garlic can be helpful to stimulate the lymphatic system, though, be sure not to use too much of it, as it can cause stomach distress in some people when not used sparingly.

- **Digestive enzymes.** Since a majority of your immune system is in your gut, if your digestion is sluggish, your body will have a harder time moving out waste. Digestive enzymes and bitters can help your body break down your food more quickly and clear out stagnant toxins that may be building up in your intestines. Some good examples are licorice root, fennel, burdock root, basil, ginger, dandelion, peppermint, cinnamon, and probiotics.

- **Green tea.** This has so many benefits! It's a potent antioxidant that prevents cell damage and also fights cancer. It's rich in polyphenols known to reduce inflammation and help your heart by increasing the level of antioxidants in the blood. It improves blood flow and is commonly used in lymphatic drainage to help with weight loss as it increases metabolism. Caffeine, which is contained in green tea, is also a major ingredient of anti-cellulite oil. The catechin compounds in green tea also help protect the neurons in the brain.

- **Zinc.** This is an invaluable element for maintaining a healthy immune system. Red meat, some seafood, poultry, beans, nuts, and whole grains provide zinc, but vegetarians may need supplementation. If your body is lacking in zinc, you may be more susceptible to getting sick, as zinc has been shown to reduce inflammation markers in the body. For that reason, medical researchers have suggested adding a zinc supplement to your arsenal in the fight against the COVID-19 virus.

Foods to Avoid

The foods on this list all promote inflammation in the body. They are also often calorie dense, adversely affect your blood sugar levels, and are low in fiber, leading to constipation and other inflammatory gut issues. In other words, they should be avoided as much as possible!

- **All processed foods, including baked goods.** These items are often high in sugar, trans fats, and/or hydrogenated fats (which can increase your risk of developing heart disease or stroke, as they raise "bad" LDL cholesterol levels, leading to narrowed and hardened arteries), sodium, and chemicals in the form of preservatives. These are not whole foods that human bodies are capable of digesting efficiently.
- **Meat, especially red meat.** This contains high levels of saturated fat as well as bacterial toxins called endotoxins. The cell walls, or lipopolysaccharides, of these endotoxins are released into the bloodstream, stimulating the immune system and triggering an inflammatory response. They can damage the intestinal wall, activating molecules that can trigger inflammatory conditions such as Crohn's disease and ulcerative colitis. If you're going to occasionally have meat, choose grass-fed and grass-finished meat when possible because it's rich in highly bioavailable iron, selenium, zinc, vitamin A, and linoleic acid (which has anti-inflammatory benefits)—and if it's organic, it won't contain the dangerous antibiotics that commercial meat does.
- **Cow's milk dairy products.** The main culprit in these is the high levels of saturated fat, which lead to the same problems as described for meat. In addition, many adults are unable to properly digest lactose, the sugar naturally found in all dairy products; when that is the case, they can experience bloating, gas, and digestive upset. Commercial

cows are also often injected with hormones, which can end up in the milk supply.

- **Sugar.** You should cut down your consumption of white sugar wherever possible. Not only does it provide no nutritional value, but any excess that you don't metabolize right away is converted to fat. Although you should also limit your intake of natural sugars if you have lymphedema or other lymphatic disorders, if you want to add some sweetness to your foods sometimes, natural sugars such as maple syrup and honey do have beneficial micronutrients that nutrient-poor refined sugars don't.

- **Gluten.** This is an inflammatory protein found in wheat, barley, and rye and most commonly found in bread, grain products, baked goods, and cereals. For some people, gluten can alter gut bacteria and function, damaging the lining of the small intestine. When this happens, your body is less able to absorb key nutrients. This is particularly important for those who are struggling with celiac disease, autoimmune disorders, diabetes, irritable bowel syndrome (IBS), and other gastrointestinal disorders.

- **Salt.** According to the American Heart Association, adults need only 1,500 milligrams per day—but the average American adult consumes more than twice that amount. Excess sodium consumption makes you retain water, which leads to bloating, puffiness, and a potential imbalance in the gut microbiome, which can trigger inflammatory conditions and is crucial to curtail if you have any lymphatic disorder.

Stay Hydrated!

As mentioned in chapter 3, a common cause of lymph congestion is dehydration. Lymph is approximately 95 percent water. Increasing the amount of water you drink will help circulate immune cells, nourish your lymph vasculature, and flush out toxins. Drinking half your body weight in ounces of clean, purified water will keep your lymphatic system hydrated and flowing smoothly. Always choose clean, filtered water, preferably alkaline when you can. If you don't have access to alkaline water, put some lemon juice into your water (when metabolized, it is high in alkalinity). I recommend starting your morning by drinking a glass of warm water with a squeeze of lemon juice in it. Keep drinking plenty of water throughout the day, especially if you're practicing lymphatic self-massage. Water will help move out debris from your tissues and increase the benefits of your lymphatic self-care routines.

ANTI-INFLAMMATORY HERBS

Certain herbs are well known for their anti-inflammatory and anti-microbial properties and their ability to increase lymphatic microcirculation and boost the immune system. Consult your doctor, a certified naturopath, an herbalist, or a specialist in Ayurveda or Chinese medicine before taking *any* herbs, and never self-diagnose.

ANTI-INFLAMMATORY HERBS

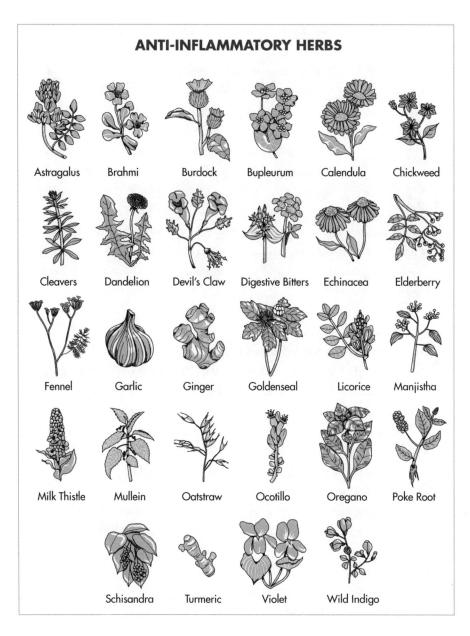

Astragalus   Brahmi   Burdock   Bupleurum   Calendula   Chickweed

Cleavers   Dandelion   Devil's Claw   Digestive Bitters   Echinacea   Elderberry

Fennel   Garlic   Ginger   Goldenseal   Licorice   Manjistha

Milk Thistle   Mullein   Oatstraw   Ocotillo   Oregano   Poke Root

Schisandra   Turmeric   Violet   Wild Indigo

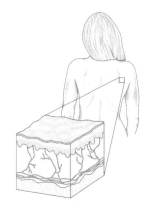

PILLAR 3: SKIN CARE AND BODY CARE

Taking proper care of your skin is essential to good lymphatic health. Your skin is the largest lymphatic organ, constantly absorbing airborne pollutants and serving as an essential line of defense against invaders. The majority of lymphatic vessels and capillaries reside just underneath its surface, where they absorb harmful chemicals and filter them through the lymphatic system. When your skin is dry or cracked, bacteria can enter and spread an infection called cellulitis, in which the lymph is stagnant. If your skin feels tight, it might be dehydrated. Drinking more fluids will nourish and bathe your cells and help to keep your lymph flowing optimally.

Nontoxic and Organic Skin Care Products Are a Must

Approximately 60 percent of what you put onto your skin is absorbed into your lymphatic system. This is why it's important to choose skin care products, as well as home cleaning products (which can get onto your hands and into your lungs), that are clean and safe.

Look for nontoxic and organic products made with as few ingredients as possible. For skin care, I recommend choosing products with a low pH, close to that of the acid mantle of your skin, which will help keep it smooth and prevent it from drying out. Using hydrating products with a pH balance of 5 or under will help protect your skin against harmful microbes, bacteria, and pollutants while still providing necessary moisture. Organic argan oil, for example, is an effective moisturizer that rarely causes irritation or toxicity. Raw organic shea butter is another excellent choice, and it's actually used as a base ingredient in many expensive skin care products.

Read labels carefully and be aware of what you're applying, especially with children's products. If you're going to use chemicals and synthetic ingredients, know what they are! Some of the chemical ingredients used in sunscreens, such as oxybenzone, were once thought to be miraculous protection against sunburn—but scientists have since discovered that they are endocrine disruptors and possibly carcinogenic, and they have been banned in many countries. Certain preservatives, such as parabens, have also been tied to certain cancers, as they are estrogen-mimicking endocrine disruptors. More than 1,400 chemicals are banned or restricted in personal care products by the European Union; in contrast, the United States bans only 49 chemicals. The US federal government hasn't updated its list since 1938! This sad truth explains why a toxic chemical such as formaldehyde is still allowed to sneak into common beauty items, including nail polish, hair straighteners, and mascara. Websites such as the Environmental Working Group (www.ewg.org) provide free databases that rate thousands of personal care products so you can make informed decisions about what to use. I highly recommend you take inventory of your medicine cabinet and bathroom shelves and make any necessary adjustments. Your lymphatic system will thank you!

The Benefits of Taking a Bath

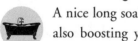 A nice long soak in a bathtub is a great way to unwind while also boosting your lymphatic system. I usually recommend my clients take an Epsom salts bath after a lymphatic massage session, as it will enhance the therapeutic effects of draining toxins. Additionally, a soak in a bath helps promote the parasympathetic nervous system, which resets the body from the harmful effects of stress.

  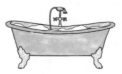

There are many bath-enhancing products out there, from oils to gels to salts to bath bombs. If you're looking to add something special to your bath, please be very careful and read the labels. I recommend Epsom salts, as they contain a compound of sulfites and magnesium that flushes toxins and heavy metals out of your body through a process called reverse osmosis. Soaking in an Epsom salts bath can reduce inflammation and improve circulation and digestion, and it couldn't be any easier to do. Sweet almond oil, calendula, and oatmeal are great ingredients for soothing the skin. And if you like a scented bath, add a few drops of a pure essential oil. Different ones contain different therapeutic properties: lavender, rose, and chamomile are particularly good for relaxation; lemon, peppermint, and rosemary help congestion; clary sage and ylang-ylang are my go-tos when I want to luxuriate and feel indulgent. When I have the time, I'll cut up slices of cucumber and grapefruit and toss them into the bath, too.

Just fill your tub with hot water, pour two heaping cups of Epsom salts into the bathtub, and let it dissolve. You may have to slide down a bit so the water can reach the lymph nodes in your neck. Sit up from time to time to give your head a break from the heat. Soak for at least twenty minutes to receive the full therapeutic value, and be sure to drink plenty of water during and after your bath. Epsom salts foot baths are terrific, too, and have been known to increase lymph circulation. Fill a bucket or large bowl with hot water, add a cup of Epsom salts, immerse your feet, and enjoy.

NOTE: Don't use Epsom salts if you're diabetic, as they can dry the skin and complicate existing foot problems. If you have lymphedema, use body-temperature water for your soak instead of hot water.

Bath Recipes

If you're looking to take your bath ritual to the next level, here are a couple of simple DIY recipes that will provide therapeutic value and feel indulgent!

Detox bath soak. Make a detox mix with two cups of Epsom salts, a half cup of apple cider vinegar, a quarter cup of baking soda (which has properties that may help remove bacteria, odors, and acidity and soothe skin irritations involving itching, swelling, and candida), and any herbs of your choice (I recommend chamomile and calendula). The acid in the apple cider vinegar will bind to toxins to help remove them from your body, and the potassium will assist in breaking up mucus and clearing the lymph nodes. Fill the tub with hot water and add your detox mix. Soak for at least fifteen to twenty minutes. Rinse in a shower afterward. This soak is particularly beneficial for athletic recovery, sore muscles, and detoxification.

Lung-clearing bath soak. Fill your tub with hot water, pour in two cups of Epsom salts, and add a few drops of eucalyptus essential oil. (If you happen to have some fresh eucalyptus leaves on hand, you can place them in the tub.) Soak for at least twenty minutes. Eucalyptus is known to relieve upper respiratory issues and is used as an ingredient in over-the-counter chest rubs. If you have sinus congestion or are otherwise looking to clear out mucus, you can hang some fresh eucalyptus leaves in the shower and steam up the room before you bathe. This will allow its medicinal properties to permeate the air.

Do-It-Yourself Face Masks

Puffiness in your face can be a sign of lymphatic congestion. In addition to the "Get Glowing Skin" sequence on page 129, a face mask can help reduce redness or tension that is constricting lymph flow. Clay masks are well known to help reduce inflammation and restore a vital glow to your skin and can be used on any part of the body. Dead Sea, lava, pumice, and bentonite clays contain an assortment of minerals, which is why estheticians use them to cleanse and restore the microbiome of the face.

Clay skin mask. Put a small amount of pure bentonite clay into a bowl. Add a scant two teaspoons of apple cider vinegar and enough water to make a smooth paste. Apply to skin and let sit for twenty minutes. You will feel your skin tighten as it dries. That's normal! Use warm water and a soft washcloth to remove the mask.

NOTE: Apple cider vinegar may cause your skin to feel hot. If you are allergic to it, do not apply it to your face. If you are unsure if you are allergic to it, you can test it on your hand first.

Glowing skin face mask. Mix one beaten egg yolk (or half an avocado, mashed), one tablespoon of honey, and one teaspoon of cacao (optional—add a dash or a quarter teaspoon of cinnamon or turmeric). Honey has wonderful antibacterial and antiviral properties that will brighten your skin. It's also great for scars and helps speed up the repair of skin cells. Egg yolk and avocado are effective moisturizers; cacao is an antioxidant. Cinnamon can help reduce acne blemishes and marks. Turmeric's active ingredient is curcumin, which has antioxidant properties to protect your skin against free-radical damage. Whisk all the ingredients in a bowl together until it forms a nice paste. Apply to your face evenly. Leave on for fifteen to twenty minutes, then wash off. You will be amazed at how clean your skin feels and how your skin glows!

NOTE: Cinnamon may cause your skin to feel hot. If you are allergic to it, do not apply it to your face. If you are unsure if you are allergic to it, you can test it on your hand first.

Dry Brushing

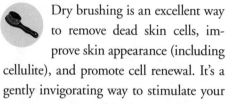 Dry brushing is an excellent way to remove dead skin cells, improve skin appearance (including cellulite), and promote cell renewal. It's a gently invigorating way to stimulate your nervous system and improve your energy, immune function, and lymph flow.

When dead cells linger on the surface of your skin, your pores can become clogged. Since your pores are one of the primary ways your skin detoxes (through sweating), clogging places an additional burden on organs such as the liver and kidneys and can undermine their proper function. Dry brushing unclogs pores and improves blood circulation, boosting your body's natural detoxification process, which improves your digestion. I recommend brushing in long, gentle strokes (not circles) to activate your lymphatic vessels. Avoid brushing too hard so as not to irritate your skin.

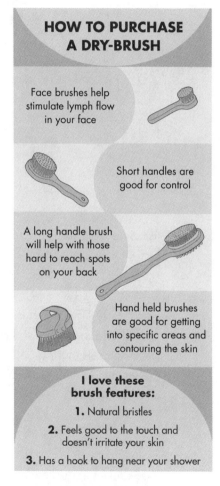

HOW TO PURCHASE A DRY-BRUSH

Face brushes help stimulate lymph flow in your face

Short handles are good for control

A long handle brush will help with those hard to reach spots on your back

Hand held brushes are good for getting into specific areas and contouring the skin

I love these brush features:

1. Natural bristles

2. Feels good to the touch and doesn't irritate your skin

3. Has a hook to hang near your shower

How to Dry-Brush

Whenever I teach dry brushing, I show people the lymphotomes, or specific regions, and the corresponding lymph nodes they need to brush toward to

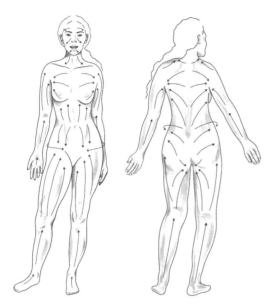

optimize results. *Massage your lymph node clusters first.* This will encourage the vacuum effect of lymphatic circulation. I recommend dry brushing two to five times a week. Shower after dry brushing to rinse off the dead cells. You can wash your brush once in a while with warm water and soap then hang it to dry. Replace the brush after one year.

NOTE: If your skin is too sensitive to dry-brush, you can use Ayurvedic silk garshana gloves, which can easily be found online. Dry brushes are available online as well as in most health food stores.

How to Dry-Brush Your Body

It's a good general rule to brush toward your heart, but here's how you can dry-brush more specifically to stimulate your lymphatic system by massaging the lymph nodes and brushing toward them. Work proximally to distally.

Step 1

Stimulate the right and left supraclavicular lymphatic nodes at the base of your neck just above your collarbone. Press your fingertips **down** into the hollows of your collarbone. Massage in a *J* motion, pressing *lightly* **down** and **out** toward your shoulders. Repeat ten times.

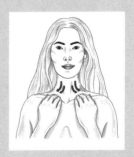

Step 2

Stimulate the axillary lymph nodes in your armpit: Place your hand in your armpit, your index finger resting *gently* in the groove of your armpit. Pulse **upward** into your armpit. Repeat ten times.

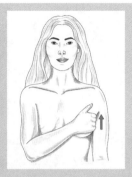

Step 3

Repeat Step 2 on your opposite armpit.

Step 4

Dry-brush from your hand up your inner and outer arm to the axillary lymph nodes in your armpit. Repeat on your opposite side.

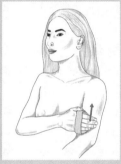

Step 5

Dry-brush your right breast into your right armpit and dry-brush your left breast into your left armpit. Then dry-brush from your sternum and middle of your chest toward your heart.

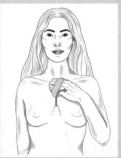

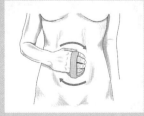

Step 6

Dry-brush your abdomen in clockwise circles; this is the direction your colon runs in and will help stimulate your digestion.

Step 7

Dry-brush your lower back and love handles toward your abdomen.

Step 8

If you have a long-handled brush with which you can reach the back of your body, brush your posterior torso and upper back toward the front of your body. The lymphatic fluid from the back of your body drains toward the front into your heart area.

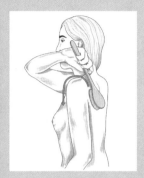

Step 9

Stimulate the inguinal lymph nodes at the top of your thigh: Place your hand on the top of your inner thigh. Massage C-strokes **upward** into the crease of your thigh. Repeat five times. Repeat on your opposite thigh.

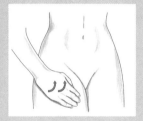

Step 10

Dry-brush from your right knee to the inguinal lymph nodes at the top of your thigh. Dry-brush above, over, and underneath your knee and up to your thigh crease. Brush your lower leg up to your thigh. Brush the back of your calves toward the front of your leg. Brush from your foot to your knee. Repeat on your left leg.

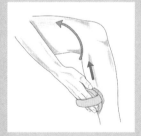

Step 11

Repeat Step 6: Dry-brush your abdomen in clockwise circles.

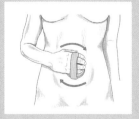

Step 12
Repeat Step 5: Dry-brush up the center of your chest.

Step 13
Dry-brush your abdomen again and brush all the way up the midline of your body to your heart.

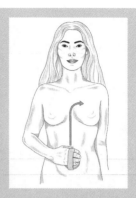

How to Dry-Brush Your Face
I recommend using a separate, softer brush for your face.

Step 1
Stimulate the lymph nodes at the base of your neck with your fingertips.

Step 2
Dry-brush from your ears down your neck to the lymph nodes at your collarbone on both sides. Repeat ten times.

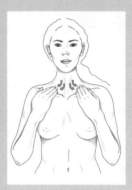

Step 3
Dry-brush your face from your chin to your ears. Repeat ten times.

Step 4
Dry-brush from your cheeks to your ears. Repeat ten times.

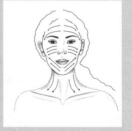

Step 5
Dry-brush up from the bridge of your nose to your forehead, then from your forehead to your temples. Repeat ten times.

Step 6
Dry-brush over your ears and down your neck. Repeat ten times.

Step 7
Repeat Step 1: Stimulate the lymph nodes at the base of your neck with your fingertips.

NOTE: Do not brush over open wounds or irritated skin.

Gua Sha and Jade Rolling

Using a gua sha stone or jade roller to remove puffiness, fine lines, and wrinkles on your face has become increasingly popular in the beauty industry over the last few years. If you've watched a how-to video, you've likely seen someone telling you to move the roller up your neck, onto your face. By now you know that that's the *opposite* of lymphatic drainage! The reason aestheticians tell you to move fluid into your face is that it brings blood and nutrients to your face, since your circulatory system moves blood from the center of your body out to your peripheries.

Lymph is different; it moves from your peripheries toward your heart. In order to drain stagnation in your face, try moving the gua sha stone or jade roller *down your neck first*. (It's the same principle as clearing your bathtub drain that you read about in "Principles of Self-Massage" in chapter 3.) I recommend massaging the right and left lymphatic nodes at your collarbone with your fingertips before using a roller or stone to prep your lymphatic circulation. You'll greatly improve your results.

Take Care of Your Nails, Too

Everyone likes to indulge in a manicure every now and then, but painting your nails isn't always the healthiest self-care ritual. Most commercial nail polishes contain the toxin formaldehyde, a preservative that has been recognized by the National Cancer Institute as a potential carcinogen—one so dangerous that it's banned in Europe. Not only does formaldehyde cause brittle nails, making them more susceptible to peeling and breaking, but it can also irritate your skin and in some cases cause an allergy. Gel manicures pose a problem as well, because most curing lamps used to dry the gel emit ultraviolet A light, which is a known cause of the kind of cellular damage that causes aging and increases the risk of skin cancer. If you're going to use polish, I suggest you find a nontoxic brand; there are many available these days. If you have a lymphatic condition such as lymphedema, you will want to take extra precautions when visiting a nail salon and avoid sharing tools with other customers. Although it might be better to place the care of your nails, especially your toenails, in the hands of a professional, you should proceed with caution when cutting the cuticles to avoid nicks that can introduce bacteria. If you have or are at risk of developing leg lymphedema, you might be best served having your toenails trimmed by a podiatrist to avoid fungal infections and to maintain proper foot hygiene. If you have or are at risk of developing arm lymphedema, it's better to bring your own tools to the nail salon and avoid cutting your cuticles. It's also a good idea to soften your cuticles with a good cuticle moisturizer, rather than cutting them, and maintain good hand hygiene.

Lymphatic Cupping

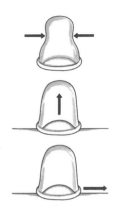

Cupping, often used as an adjunct to acupuncture, is a therapy that uses small, bulblike suction cups—placed on various meridian points—to treat sore muscles, improve blood flow, and promote relaxation.

Lymphatic cupping utilizes a similar concept but differs in that you will move the cups continually on your body instead of leaving them on your skin in one place for a long time. Lymphatic cupping won't leave the circular bruise on the skin that's synonymous with traditional cupping. Although those bruises are okay for acupuncture, we want to avoid that effect in lymphatic self-care as it can bring more inflammation to the area and potentially create an adverse lymph effect.

During lymphatic cupping, you'll move the cups superficially along the body's pattern of drainage toward your lymph nodes. The cups lift the excess fluid that is right under your skin to create a suction or vacuum effect on your tissues. This procedure will give you the famous waist and thigh contour shaping you see in beauty magazines because it reduces inflammation.

You can purchase suction cups online and use them at home. The cups come in various sizes to use on your body and your face.

How to Do Lymphatic Cupping

Step 1

With your hands, stimulate the lymph nodes that drain the region you will be working on. For instance, if you are cupping your legs, massage the inguinal lymph nodes in the thigh crease at the top of your thigh; if you are cupping your face, stimulate the lymph nodes near your collarbones. I also suggest doing deep diaphragmatic breathing to stimulate lymph flow from your lower extremities.

Step 2
Apply some oil or lotion to your skin.

Step 3
If you have a rubber suction cup, first squeeze the cup; this pulls the air out of the cup before you put it on your skin. Once the cup is on your skin, release it. The cup will gently pull the skin, creating a lifting or suction feeling. Hold the cup there for two seconds, then glide it in a straight line toward the nearest lymph nodes. Repeat ten times per line.

Step 4
Work in zones. For example, cup your leg up the inside of your thigh ten times, then cup the middle of your leg ten times, then the outer thigh. Move the cup in long, fluid strokes, pulling the skin upward carefully as you go. Make sure you squeeze the cup each time before you put it on your skin; this is how to get the optimal stretch of skin and avoid gliding. Work from proximal to distal; that is, work on your upper thigh before working on your lower leg. If you want to concentrate on a particular area (one that has cellulite, for example) feel free to spend a few more minutes there using shorter, smaller movements.

If you are using a cup on your face, work in lines from your chin to your ear, your cheeks to your ears, your forehead to your ears, and from your ears down your neck to the right and left lymphatic nodes at the base of your neck near your collarbone.

Step 5
To finish, stimulate your lymph nodes with your hands again.

Reflexology

Reflexology is an ancient practice that uses a system of energy transmission by applying pressure to specific locations on your feet, hands, or ears to clear blockages and restore vitality throughout the body. Take a look at the reflexology map below, which shows you the location of all your organs and the corresponding pressure points. It also shows you the localized lymphatic stimulating points.

I first studied this modality in the early 1990s in massage school, and it felt like magic. By massaging specific points on your feet, you can alleviate tension, pain, and stress; clear stagnant toxins and improve your digestion; and calm your anxiety and improve your mood.

We expect so much from our feet; they hold our weight all day long, with little care paid to them aside from a little toenail painting once in a while. It's common to experience painful areas on your feet. Use more

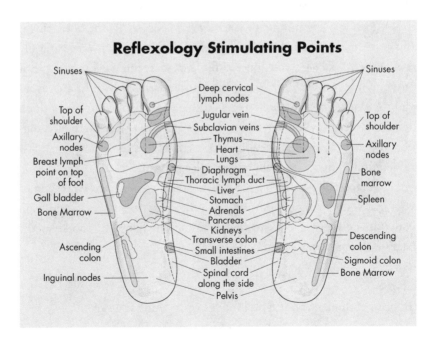

Reflexology Stimulating Points

pressure than during your typical self-massage sequence to break up any knots you find. Begin slowly, and work the pressure up bit by bit.

This sequence is designed to boost your lymphatic system, specifically targeting your lymphatic and digestive reflex points in your body.

How to Do Reflexology
Once you understand the reflexology map, you're ready to begin.

Step 1
Make sure your hands and feet are thoroughly clean.

Step 2
I recommend sitting comfortably. With your right hand, brush the top of your right foot from the base of your toes toward the top of your ankle. These are reflex zones for lymph. Repeat ten times.

Step 3
Place the palms of both hands on either side of your right ankle. Flex and point your foot while massaging the fluid from your ankle up toward your leg. This is the reflex point for the genital areas. It is often the first area to get swollen when you fly. *Gently* massage C-strokes over the built-up fluid as you flex and point your foot. Repeat ten times.

Step 4
Place the palm of your hand under the instep of your foot. Rotate your foot in both directions while massaging the center of the bottom of your foot. This warms up your digestion organ reflex points. Repeat ten times.

Step 5

The top of the foot between the big toe and second toe is a wonderful lymphatic reflex point for your breasts. With your fingers, massage from the webbing of your big toe to the top of your ankle, slowly pressing **in** and **up**. Notice if you have any soreness or tension here. Spend some time delicately massaging C-strokes until the pain has subsided. Repeat at least ten times. Then massage the top of your foot from the webbing to the ankle. Repeat ten times.

Step 6

Referring to the reflexology map, massage the remaining points on your foot to circulate lymph.

- Massage the colon point on both feet to stimulate digestion; the ascending, transverse, descending, sigmoid colon, and small intestine points to promote elimination. This will stimulate the cisterna chyli and thoracic duct.
- Massage the spleen and kidney points.
- Massage the diaphragm points to open your lungs.
- Massage along the insides of your feet; those are the points for your spinal cord, which will help to melt tension and induce the rest-and-digest parasympathetic nervous system response.
- Massage the arm, axillary nodes, and breast points again.

Step 7

Repeat on the opposite foot.

NOTE: If you're pregnant, do not press on the ovary point or thumb web. Check with your practitioner prior to doing any reflexology self-treatments. If you have lymphedema, work *very lightly*.

Create Your Own Reflexology Record

If you want to keep a record of your tender spots, all you need to do is get a blank piece of paper and draw the outlines of your feet on it. Label each foot. Add the date. As you massage your feet, mark an **X** on the paper where you're sore.

When I do this, sometimes there are so many tender spots I can't remember them all, so I'm glad I've written them down. This map will also serve as your guide to exploring other lymphatic self-massage sequences in chapter 4 for extra clearing. During any body work, you may experience a range of emotions. Let them be reminders to tend to your inner landscape.

Castor Oil Packs

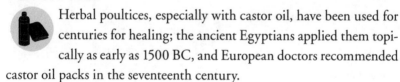 Herbal poultices, especially with castor oil, have been used for centuries for healing; the ancient Egyptians applied them topically as early as 1500 BC, and European doctors recommended castor oil packs in the seventeenth century.

Castor oil (*Ricinus communis*) comes from the castor bean, which is native to India, Africa, and the Mediterranean. It is extremely high in health-promoting ricinoleic acid, which has a chemical structure similar to the prostaglandins in our bodies that reduce inflammation. It's long been used as a laxative, wound healer, and immune-boosting remedy.

Using castor oil packs became popular again in the twentieth century after a double-blind study done by Harvey Grady, who reported in the *Journal of Naturopathic Medicine* that the use of castor oil packs enhanced immunological function. Many doctors now acknowledge the efficacy of castor oil packs for many different conditions. Castor oil's

298 THE BOOK OF LYMPH

anti-inflammatory and antimicrobial properties have been shown to provide the following benefits:

- Improves lymphatic circulation
- Balances stomach acid by stimulating liver, gallbladder, and pancreas secretions
- Improves constipation by stimulating peristalsis of the gastrointestinal and urinary organs, and reducing bloating and alleviating cramps
- Improves skin conditions, headaches, and PMS symptoms, as well as breast and ovarian cysts
- Increases immune-fighting T cells
- Regulates metabolism and heals tissues and organs such as the liver, gallbladder, uterus, and other reproductive organs
- Stimulates the parasympathetic rest-and-digest response

How to Make a Castor Oil Pack

You will need a folded-up yard of cotton or wool flannel (preferably undyed and unbleached), a sheet of plastic cut slightly larger than the flannel to catch any drips, castor oil, a heating pad or hot water bottle, and a container to store everything in after use.

Step 1

Preheat the heating pad or hot water bottle. Place the flannel over the plastic sheet in a sink in your bathroom or kitchen (in case the oil drips) and saturate the flannel in castor oil.

Step 2

Lie down somewhere comfortable and place the castor oil pack on top of the warm heating pad or hot water bottle. Apply it to your skin with the cloth side down onto your abdomen, over your liver, gallbladder, or chest.

Step 3

Leave the pack on for forty-five minutes to one hour.

Step 4

Clean your skin with warm water in which you have dissolved a few teaspoons of baking soda (its alkalinity will neutralize the acidic toxins that have been pulled out of your body). Turn off the heating pad or empty the hot water bottle and store your castor oil pack in a container in the fridge.

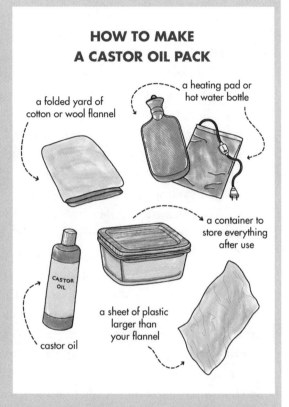

HOW TO MAKE A CASTOR OIL PACK

a folded yard of cotton or wool flannel

a heating pad or hot water bottle

a container to store everything after use

CASTOR OIL

a sheet of plastic larger than your flannel

castor oil

You can try using castor oil packs three times a week for three weeks, followed by one week off. Other recommendations include three days on, three days off. Replace the pack if you've been sick or after a few months of regular use.

NOTE: For topical application only. Do not ingest. Some health food stores sell castor oil packs, and you can even find a castor oil pack holder that comes with two Velcro strips that secure the flannel over your abdomen, along with a pouch to hold your heating pad in place so you don't have to use plastic.

Infrared Biomats, Blankets, Saunas, and Lasers and Light Therapy

Infrared Biomats and Blankets

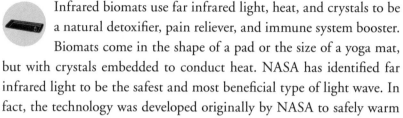 Infrared biomats use far infrared light, heat, and crystals to be a natural detoxifier, pain reliever, and immune system booster.

Biomats come in the shape of a pad or the size of a yoga mat, but with crystals embedded to conduct heat. NASA has identified far infrared light to be the safest and most beneficial type of light wave. In fact, the technology was developed originally by NASA to safely warm space stations and space vehicles.

An infrared biomat is different from a heating pad in that it doesn't contain heating coils that can hurt your skin. It has electromagnetic field (EMF) protection built in. The technology combines deep-penetrating infrared rays along with negative ions that transfer radiant heat evenly through the body as far down as the molecular level. Infrared biomats provide natural pain relief and deep relaxation. Not only are they de-toxifiers, they also relax muscles, reduce pain and stiffness, and improve circulation. If you are someone who has a hard time sleeping, I encour-age you to invest in a biomat; they cost several hundred dollars and up, but many of my clients tell me that the investment is worth it, as it helps alleviate muscle tension within fifteen minutes and has enabled them to sleep better. My clients who have tried one have called it a game changer and say they can't live without it.

If you are concerned that heat is contraindicated to your condition, you can set the biomat to low so it doesn't go above your body tempera-ture. I love using them, but the advanced models can be pricey! Many spas and other businesses are now offering infrared saunas and biomats as services so you can experience this modality for a nominal fee.

Infrared Saunas

Sweat rituals are found in many cultures. Sweating helps the body rid itself of toxins, which will improve your digestion as well as your complexion. Some gyms and salons have infrared saunas, which look the same as regular dry-heat saunas but use invisible far-infrared light, as it has far less energy (15 micrometers to 2 millimeters) than does visible light (400 to 750 nanometers) but a host of benefits.

Far-infrared light penetrates the surface of the skin down to the cellular level, which can lower your blood temperature, give your skin a glow, and aid in weight loss, because you can reportedly burn up to 600 calories in just thirty minutes in an infrared sauna. These saunas also help with detoxification, pain relief, and the production of collagen and white blood cells. And because they need to be well ventilated to allow stale air to exit the sauna, infrared saunas are much more comfortable to sit in for longer periods of time than conventional saunas are. You won't experience difficulty breathing or become extremely overheated as you might in a conventional sauna.

Infrared Lasers

Using the same infrared technology, personal lasers are being introduced to the lymphatic community and have been approved by the FDA for people with lymphedema to reduce inflammation and swelling. The lasers create a photochemical reaction at a cellular level that penetrates the tissue and influences the cellular metabolic process, which helps promote blood and lymph flow. The laser is used to help heal skin wounds, athletic injuries, muscle soreness, and sprained ligaments.

NOTE: If you are at risk of developing lymphedema or lymphatic pooling, consult with your lymphatic therapist to see if saunas and lasers are safe for your condition.

Light Therapy

Light therapy is gaining interest among lymphatic health seekers. It's a noninvasive technology that uses electrical signals and negatively charged light photons at low currents to stimulate the release of bonded proteins and other binding agents that cause swelling and blockages in cell clusters. Light therapy uses specific wavelengths to correct cells' out-of-balance electromagnetic charge. It's reported to release built-up fluids, enabling them to move through lymphatic pathways more easily.

The theory behind this therapy is that lymphatic protein interactions are primarily electrical. You may have heard of a color light therapy called chromotherapy, which has seven colors in its spectrum. Some spas offer this technology when you get a facial, as the red, purple, or blue light masks are used to cleanse the microbiome of the face and reduce the bacteria that cause acne. Many companies are using the technology in self-care tools to help reverse inflammation in the body. The other colors in the spectrum provide different benefits that work on varying energy points to balance the body—green is calming, yellow soothes inflammation, orange is revitalizing to dull skin—and restore mental and physical health, not just to the face but throughout the body.

Knowing what you do now about the pulsing mechanism of lymphangions, this concept makes some sense. Researchers are investigating the therapeutic benefits of light therapy for healing wounds, neurodegenerative disorders, reducing inflammation, healing muscle injuries, and dealing with other conditions to prove its efficacy.

NOTE: If you have lymphedema, please consult a Certified Lymphedema Therapist to determine if this is the right application for you. I do not recommend it as a replacement for manual lymphatic drainage or CDT.

MEDITATION: A THROUGH LINE OF EVERY PILLAR

Countless studies have proven that meditation can reduce stress levels. Doctors will tell you that reducing your stress is one of the most important changes you can make to improve your health. It's right up there with diet, exercise, and sleep! I was first introduced to meditation when I was just shy of eleven years old. It's long been a calming resource that I can use any time I feel overwhelmed, out of control, or in pain. I came to rely on my meditation practice like an old friend, allowing me to access a deeper part of myself where I believed that everything would be okay—even if it didn't seem that way in the moment.

Over the years, I've studied many forms of meditation, including at Zen centers and silent Vipassana retreats. Each experience gave me tools to remain calm in spite of the murky waters of my mind. Meditation triggers the functions of the parasympathetic nervous system, which enables healing to occur. When you meditate, you move from shallow chest breathing into deeper diaphragmatic breathing, which improves your lymph circulation. Developing a way to relax your mind, your nerves, and your emotions will reduce your stress and improve your health in the long term. If you've ever taken a breath work class or been curious about it, the benefits are endless! Not only will it improve your mood and sleep, but deep breathing is a proven way to stimulate lymphatic flow. That's why I developed a "Deep Diaphragmatic Breathing" sequence (page 116) to accompany the "Heart and Lung Opener" and "Abdominal Massage" sequences on pages 173 and 122.

How to Do a Simple Meditation/Creative Visualization

I learned this technique when I was a child and my mother was battling lung cancer. One of our family friends was a Silva Method meditation teacher, and he came by the house a few times to teach us how to meditate—or "go to level," as he called it. His technique was quite simple, as you'll see below. First he made sure we were seated comfortably (lying down is okay, too). Then he instructed us to count backward and recite a few calming words. Next he had us visualize a healing space in our minds. He told us to pick a place in nature—or somewhere else where we felt safe and happy—and taught us to envelop the space with soothing symbols, images, and objects that made us feel as though we were in a dream home. Each session lasted only about fifteen minutes, but I felt as though I traveled deeply into myself to a place within me that was pure.

It wasn't until I was much older that I realized that that meditation had been designed to introduce us to a deeper state of consciousness— and create a unique room to serve as a safe harbor in our minds. Now, more than three decades later, I still visit that same place when I need some solace. I don't think I appreciated the value of learning to access the deepest part of myself until I was much older. Having that training early on provided me with an inner strength and ability to access my intuition. I've meditated in emergency room hospital beds, prayed for the health of a loved one, and visited my imaginary sanctuary in times when I feel out of sorts or out of control. It always makes me feel grounded and serene.

I've been "going to level" to the same place in my mind since I was a young girl. The room feels rich with sacred healing powers and protection. The space you create for yourself will become your own. You don't need to tell anyone about it. I don't think I've ever shared the details of mine with anyone—except maybe my brother, because we told each other everything when we were young. The sequence below will show you how to cultivate your own slice of Heaven that you can cherish forever.

If you're feeling anxious, you can use this meditation while you prac- tice a self-massage sequence and send yourself unconditional love. My hope is for you to create a healing center that you can access no matter where you are.

Step 1

Begin by sitting or lying down comfortably.

Step 2

Close your eyes.

Step 3

Take a few deep breaths in and out.

Step 4

Relax the muscles of your face, jaw, and throat.

Step 5

Start counting backward from ten. When you get to nine, say to yourself, "Going deeper and deeper, into a healthier level of mind." Eight, seven, "Deeper and deeper." Six, five, "Going deeper and deeper into a healthier level of mind." Four, three, "Deeper and deeper." Two, one.

Step 6

At one, imagine you are standing at the top of a steep staircase. The staircase can be anywhere you want—a field of lavender, a snow-covered mountain peak, a sand dune leading to a soft beach. You get my point. Take the steps downward saying to yourself, "I am in a deeper, healthier state of mind."

Step 7

Visualize your ideal healing space, the sanctuary of your dreams. Walk into it. . . . What colors do you see? What sounds do you hear? What images appear? Are there windows looking onto a rain forest or at mountains? . . . Are you in a desert with blooming cacti? . . . Are there paintings on the wall . . . pictures of loved ones? . . . Are the walls arched like an adobe in New Mexico? . . . Is the ceiling an A-frame like a modern farmhouse? . . . Is it a log cabin or a glass house over the ocean? Maybe the sun is shining and there's a slight breeze in the air. Maybe you see rain pattering down or a fresh snowfall, a full moon, and a sea of stars across the sky.

Fill in the details that surround you with happy feelings. Spend some time on those details and create your magical dream office. Maybe it's your own backyard, or a resort you've seen in a magazine that's your dream vacation spot. Take time with the details. This is going to be your spot forever, so make it magnificent. How do you enter your office? Through a secret garden, a waterslide, a carousel, a zip line?

Step 8

Once you arrive in your healing sanctuary, imagine yourself—or someone you want to send healing energy to. When I was younger, I used to visualize the healthy cells in my mother's body multiplying and destroying the cancer cells. Later, when I found myself in a hospital with a dangerous dog bite, I envisioned my incision healing from the inside out and that the medication I was given was protecting me from any possible systemic infection. I've also sent healing to my uncle when he was in his last stages of life, so that he might have an easy, pain-free crossing over. Whether you are looking for some calm before a public speaking event or desiring to spread light and prayers to a loved one, your healing sanctuary is a safe, supportive place to visualize your dreams.

Step 9

When you're ready to come out of your office, count from one to three, saying "One—when I wake up, I will feel better than before. Two—I will be wide awake, in perfect health, feeling better than before. Three—better and better."

PILLAR 4: COMPRESSION

Compression is all too familiar to lymphedema patients. In the past decade, however, compression garments have become increasingly high tech, and new options have been developed to aid athletic recovery, manage mild edema (swelling), and target weight loss and even for pregnant women when they fly.

Compression bandages and garments are extremely helpful for lymph flow and are a pillar of Complete Decongestive Therapy (CDT) in mitigating lymphedema. Many people can also benefit from wearing compression socks to aid recovery from a sprain or after an elective surgery. These can also be helpful if your job requires you to stand on your feet all day. Compression socks are especially useful for airplane travel, in particular if you are older and nonambulatory and/or you are at risk of developing blood clots.

Some compression garments contain antimicrobial material, and some leggings use MicroPerle massage beads to provide an extra boost of compression to propel lymph, whether you're working out or just running errands. Medical-grade garments use a type of material called inelastic so your circulation is not cut off. It allows your muscles to contract and relax—to move with you and rest with you—which is the motion necessary to propel lymph. If you swell in the heat or due to lymphedema, you are a prime candidate to learn about medical-grade compression stockings or sleeves.

Compression pneumatic pumps are often used in CDT to treat lymphedema. They are identifiable by having multiple chambers that inflate one after the other to stimulate the flow of lymph in the right direction, from distal to proximal. You will want to work with a lymphedema therapist to make sure you are using it correctly and to find the one that's best for you. A lymphedema therapist can make sure you have the correct paperwork to determine if it's covered by your insurance because they are expensive.

There's also another type of pump, commonly referred to as a compression therapy pump. It looks like a sleeping bag that fits over your legs and abdomen or arm and chest. Originally developed to help lymphedema patients, these devices are making their way to the wellness world for their anti-inflammatory benefits and enhancements to athletic performance. This kind of pump provides gentle pulses to the body that mimic lymphatic propulsion. Although they are pricey to purchase, you might be able to find a spa or wellness center near you where you can try one out.

Kinesio Taping or Kinesiology Taping

Kinesiology taping is a rehabilitation method to assist the reduction of swelling and can accelerate lymph flow once an area has been inflamed. The specialized tape provides support and stability to muscles and joints while allowing range of motion. Using the tape in particular directions can improve lymphatic drainage because it lifts the skin microscopically. The lift and stretch of the skin (similar to what occurs during your self-massage strokes) allows the interstitial fluid to flow more freely. Applying the tape in *I*, *X*, and *Y* patterns can promote circulation, reduce pain, and restore fluid balance.

I recommend that you work with a physical therapist, occupational therapist, or lymphatic professional to learn this technique.

PILLAR 5: EXERCISE

We all know the importance of exercise to our cardiovascular system. By now you know that your lymphatic system is your second circulatory system. Lymph depends on muscle movement to move lymphatic fluid and toxins, which is why regular exercise is a natural lymph flush. The more you move your body, the more your muscle contractions will create an intrinsic, systemic lymphatic response.

The following exercises are especially useful to accompany your lymphatic self-massage practice.

Biking

 SoulCycle and Peloton turned indoor biking into a phenomenon. Biking, whether indoors or outdoors, is great because it focuses on your core and legs, two of the trickiest spots in which to encourage lymph circulation. I have clients well into their eighties who still get onto a stationary bike to strengthen their muscles and their immunity. Whether you take to the hills or follow an instructor at a gym or online, this is a sure way to enhance your lymphatic circulation.

Dancing

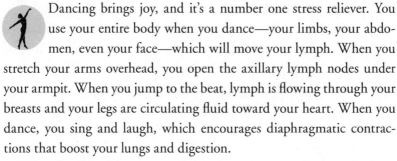 Dancing brings joy, and it's a number one stress reliever. You use your entire body when you dance—your limbs, your abdomen, even your face—which will move your lymph. When you stretch your arms overhead, you open the axillary lymph nodes under your armpit. When you jump to the beat, lymph is flowing through your breasts and your legs are circulating fluid toward your heart. When you dance, you sing and laugh, which encourages diaphragmatic contractions that boost your lungs and digestion.

What I've found in my practice is that when my clients embark on regular lymphatic self-care, they also tend to their emotional landscape by incorporating more joy and self-love in their lives. I believe that dancing and laughing are the quickest ways to inject a little (or a lot!) of joy and love into your entire being. Also, the hormone oxytocin is released when you're socializing—which is even more incentive to go dancing!

Pilates

 The inventor of the Pilates method of exercise, Joseph Pilates, initially called it Contrology. He believed that by cultivating strength with anatomical precision, you could restore health in the body. His exercises use the power of breath with all the muscle groups, especially your core, to activate every system and every cell. He developed it to improve physical strength, flexibility, and posture and to enhance mental awareness.

For the past five years, my private practice has been located in a Pilates studio. Many of my clients work with my colleagues to help decrease inflammation safely, and I've seen the results firsthand. Although there are specific exercises that increase lymph flow, as with yoga, doing an entire Pilates mat class will help wring out the stagnant toxins built up in your tissues.

Rebounding and Trampolines

 Rebounding is fantastic for your lymphatic system because it serves as a pump against gravity to propel lymph up toward your heart, which helps flush out toxins and bacteria. It's one of my favorite ways to exercise for good lymphatic health.

When you are on a rebounder, your body is always working to balance itself, which engages your core and helps your alignment as nearly every muscle group is involved. You'll burn extra calories and improve your brain's neural connections while you give your lymph the jolt it needs for that immune-boosting function. Since it's nonimpact, rebounding is also much easier on your joints than running, especially on pavement, and can prevent bone density loss. As with swimming, you will feel your lung capacity increase, too. You need to bounce for only five to ten minutes to have lasting effects on cardiovascular function and strength building. It's a fun way to burn fat and increase energy. Even my kids love it!

If you don't have room for a trampoline or rebounder, jumping rope is also great for moving your lymph.

Swimming

All of us in the lymphatic community agree that swimming is one of the best exercises for your lymphatic system because the water pressure acts like a compressor to create the perfect pump to your lymphatic vessels. Water is eight hundred times as dense as air. That compression stimulates the lymphangions to elicit the angiomotoricity response you learned about in chapter 1 to pump lymph throughout your body. Not only does swimming burn calories efficiently, it works all your major muscle groups—arms, legs, glutes, and core—at once. Swimming also helps boost circulation, flush out toxins, and decrease inflammation, all while having no impact on your joints, making it a good form of low-intensity exercise postinjury. Like rebounding, swimming will increase your lung capacity and can build bone density. If you can swim in the ocean or in a saltwater pool, even better; the salt makes the water more buoyant, and there aren't as many toxins as in chlorinated pools.

I hear from clients all the time that their swelling decreases dramatically when they swim regularly. Most community pools offer aquatic exercise classes, and there are also downloadable digital fluid-running programs (using waterproof earbuds) that you can use while you swim.

Tai Chi and Qigong

Often described as "meditation in motion," tai chi is an ancient mind-body practice based on martial arts to calm and center the mind while strengthening the body. The fluid movements connect your body to your breath. My massage teacher taught me to use this practice as a tool to keep my body grounded and aligned while maintaining a physically demanding profession. Because it's low impact, tai chi can be done at any age. It's been very beneficial for cancer clients during their grueling treatments as it helps alleviate stress and anxiety.

My teacher also taught us qigong; the translation is "vital energy cultivation" or "mastery of your energy." The movements are also slow and specific to address healing (for yourself as well as for others) through controlled breathing and movement. Cultivating either or both of these practices will be beneficial as they're a gentle and wonderful way to connect with your inner self-healer.

Vibration Plates

You may have seen vibration plates in your gym in various sizes and with various attributes: some oscillate, some pivot, some move up and down, and others do a combination of movements. They are used in combination with exercise. Research shows that they are beneficial in slowing fat accumulation, increasing metabolism, and alleviating fatigue. They oxygenate the muscles and help improve balance. Vibration plates are also a safe low-impact exercise for lymphedema patients when used on a low speed, which is why some Certified Lymphedema Therapists use them in their treatments and recommend them in our community.

When you work out on a vibration plate, it stimulates your blood flow and your lymphatic circulation as it increases the pumping action of your lymphatic vessels. It's a safe way to build bone density without the risk of musculoskeletal injury often caused by high-impact exercise. They're often used in athletic settings for the serotonin boost and neurological benefits.

Walking

Walking will always be one of the easiest ways to bring movement into your life. Any time you take a walk, you oxygenate your lungs, pump your lymphatic system, and bring joy, connectivity, creativity, and perspective to your life.

Walking is a gentle way to move your lymph without being hard on your joints. Now that you know that the main lymph drains are located in the hinges of the body, think about the ergonomics of what happens when you walk. You're swinging your arms, which stimulates the nodes under your armpits; you're propelling lymph by using your legs and your thighs; and your neck is turning from one side to the other to enjoy the view.

Walking can be done at any age. I've had clients going through cancer treatment who say all they have the energy for is to walk around their block. I tell them that that's fantastic because they are boosting their lymphatic circulation and improving their immunity at the same time.

Walking for Good Lymph Health

I once had a client who was eighty-six years old and had developed swelling in her ankles seemingly out of nowhere. After some inquiries about when she had first noticed the onset of her symptoms, she told me her dog had recently died, so she had stopped walking three times a day. I told her that when we age, the walls of our veins can collapse and make it more difficult for lymph to move up the body. The simple act of walking less had contributed to lymphatic pooling in this woman. Once she learned some simple lymphatic self-massage tips and resumed her walking routine, her swelling subsided.

Weight Training

It is a physiological fact that smooth muscle contractions, which work your muscles when you do weight training, pump lymphatic fluid. Researchers have also discovered that weight training is beneficial for people with lymphedema, lipedema, and cellulite because it decreases fat cells and may also drain excess lymphatic fluid from the area. Way back when I first started working as a lymphedema therapist, the guideline for people at risk of developing lymphedema was that they shouldn't lift more than five pounds. That recommendation has changed in the past few decades. New research shows that weight training doesn't necessarily increase fluid limb volume, meaning that supervised weight training has positive results.

Starting slow is key so you don't overwhelm your body with a buildup of uric acid or inflammation. Resistance bands and TheraBands are a great low-impact way to build bone density with resistance without fear of creating a repetitive strain injury. If you are at risk of developing lymphedema, I suggest working with a lymphedema therapist to develop a program that's safe for you.

Yoga

I've taught yoga for more than twenty years and have been practicing it for thirty. It is one of my favorite forms of exercise for the lymphatic system because it utilizes the entire muscle network, increasing the lymphatic pumping through the one-way vessels. There are also specific poses for lymph movement; inversions, for example, encourage lymph flow back to the heart, and twists move lymph through the abdomen. Pranayama breathing is similar to the "Deep Diaphragmatic Breathing" sequence on page 116 that helps improve lung capacity and digestion. But really, all yoga sequences will get your lymph flowing!

There are many ways to modify your yoga practice to support you through adverse health conditions, the aging process, and your state of mind. I often say that lymphatic drainage is akin to yoga. Many people initially try it out for the cosmetic benefits—but they stay because it transforms their health and improves their well-being in so many other ways.

IN CLOSING . . .

The ceaselessly flowing rivers of lymph are incredibly powerful in their ability to cleanse the body of toxins and waste and promote healthy immune function. What has always excited me about the field of lymphatic health is how it continuously provides new ways for people to connect to themselves and their emotions in a meaningful manner. When you feel the shifts in your energy and your mood and the freedom and lightness in your limbs, that's the aquarium of fluidity you've cultivated and that you have access to anytime and anywhere.

I hope that you will continue to use this book as a road map to create optimal health and harmony in your mind, body, and spirit. It's my greatest pleasure to share these ingredients for lymphatic health so that your journey to wellness may be a joyful and vibrant one.

In good lymphatic health always,
Lisa

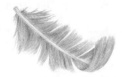

RESOURCES

HOW TO FIND A LYMPHATIC DRAINAGE TREATMENT TO SUIT YOUR GOALS

If you have lymphedema due to genetics or a secondary cause such as cancer treatment, surgery, or another condition that puts you at risk of developing lymphatic disease, you'll want to work with a Certified Lymphedema Therapist.

- Look for someone who uses the acronyms CLT (Certified Lymphedema Therapist) and CDT (Complete Decongestive Therapy). CDT is the gold standard for people with lymphedema.
- Only therapists with an MLD (Manual Lymphatic Drainage) certification can use this acronym.
- Lymphedema surgeons: The area of surgery for lymphedema patients has blossomed in the past decade. Most surgeons work with lymphedema therapists and are a good resource to help you navigate your options. You can search for one through the LE&RN website listed below.

THESE NONPROFITS LIST MLD AND CDT THERAPIST REFERRALS ON THEIR WEBSITES

International Lymphoedema
Framework
https://www.lympho.org
Lymphatic Education & Resource
Network (LE&RN)
https://lymphaticnetwork.org

Lymphology Association of North
America (LANA)
https://www.clt-lana.org
National Lymphedema Network
(NLN)
https://lymphnet.org

THESE SCHOOLS CERTIFY IN LYMPHEDEMA THERAPY AND HAVE THERAPIST REFERRAL NETWORKS

Academy of Lymphatic Studies
https://www.acols.com
Casley-Smith International (C-SI)
http://www.casleysmithinternational.org/
Chikly Health Institute
https://chiklyinstitute.com

Dr. Vodder School International
https://vodderschool.com
Foeldi College
https://www.foeldicollege.com
Klose Training & Consulting
https://klosetraining.com
Norton School of Lymphatic Therapy
https://www.nortonschool.com

HOW TO FIND A COMPRESSION FITTER

If you're in need of medical-grade compression garments, bandages, or a pneumatic pump, you will want to work with a Certified Lymphedema Therapist or Certified Garment Fitter. Most schools listed above that certify lymphedema therapists have resources to help you find compression garments and fitters.

Some companies have off-the-shelf garments available to purchase online without a fitter. Or you can order a custom-fit garment if your limb or body part doesn't fit into an off-the-shelf garment. Your lymphedema therapist can help you obtain one specifically tailored to your needs.

NOTE: An improperly fitted sleeve or glove can make lymphedema worse by placing too much or too little pressure on certain areas of your limb, causing fluid to back up and worsen your condition. In addition to therapists, some medical supply companies have certified fitters who will take measurements of your arm, hand, legs, or other areas to select the best garment for you.

These companies provide medical-grade compression garments:

Amoena
https://www.amoena.com/us-en
JoviPak
https://jovipak.com/upper-body/bellisse.htm
Jobst USA
https://www.jobst-usa.com

Juzo
http://www.juzousa.com
LympheDIVAs
https://lymphedivas.com
Medi USA
https://www.mediusa.com
Solaris
http://solarismed.com

GLOSSARY OF LYMPH TERMS

ANASTOMOSIS: The connection between the lymphatic vessels used in lymphatic massage to move fluid from a congested body part to a healthier-functioning region. For example, the interaxillary anastomosis moves fluid across the chest.

ATLAS OF LYMPH: A drainage map of the lymphatic system of the body.

AXILLARY LYMPH NODES: The lymph nodes in the armpits that drain a majority of the arm, breast, and upper torso.

CHYLE: Liquid fat products characterized by a cloudy, milky white color that are created after you digest dietary fat. Chyle is absorbed into the lymphatic vessels in the small intestine. It is characterized by a cloudy, milky white color.

CISTERNA CHYLI: A sac that absorbs fat from the small intestines that gives lymph its milky white color. The beginning of the thoracic duct.

COMPLETE DECONGESTIVE THERAPY (CDT): The medically approved treatment for lymphedema developed by Drs. Michael and Ethel Földi. Treatment includes manual lymphatic drainage (MLD), compression bandaging and garments, exercise, skin and nail care, and self-care.

COMPRESSION GARMENTS: Garments for limbs and other body parts that use gradient pressure to reduce swelling and encourage lymph flow.

CUBITAL LYMPH NODES: Also called the epitrochlear lymph nodes; located in the elbow crease that drains some of the lymphatic fluid from the lower arm, hand, and fingers.

DEEPER LYMPHATIC NETWORK: Deeper regions of your body such as trunks and ducts that are responsible for returning filtered lymph to your blood circulation at the junction of the internal jugular vein and subclavian vein.

EDEMA: Swelling categorized by low protein levels in fluid.

FUNCTIONAL RESERVE: The relationship between the lymph load and transport capacity that enables the lymphatic system to respond to an increase in lymph volume by increasing the lymph transport ability.

GLYMPHATIC SYSTEM: The network of lymphatic vessels in the brain that eliminate waste using cerebrospinal fluid.

GUT-ASSOCIATED LYMPHOID TISSUE (GALT): Consists of Peyer's patches, isolated lymphoid follicles, and mesenteric lymph nodes.

INGUINAL LYMPH NODES: The cluster of lymph nodes at the top of the thigh in the thigh crease that drains lymphatic fluid from the legs, superficial areas of the lower abdomen, and pelvic cavity.

INTERSTITIAL FLUID: The fluid space between your cells.

LACTEALS: Lacteals merge to form larger lymphatic vessels which transport chyle to the thoracic duct where it then joins the bloodstream.

LIPEDEMA: A genetic condition caused by irregular deposits of fat in the body, which can block lymphatic vessels.

LUMBAR LYMPH NODES: Located between the diaphragm and the pelvis, these lymph nodes drain the pelvic organs and abdominal wall.

LYMPH/LYMPHATIC FLUID: Water, white blood cells, cellular waste, excess protein, pathogens, and fat that the lymphatic system absorbs from the interstitial space.

LYMPH LOAD: Substances in the lymph that are removed by the lymphatic system, such as metabolic waste, cellular debris, proteins, hormones, fat-soluble vitamins, and immune cells

LYMPH NODES: Filtering stations in the body that store white blood cells and filter impurities and pathogens from the interstitial fluid.

LYMPH TIME VOLUME: The amount of lymph that can be transported in a unit of time. It's lower when the body is at rest and higher during activity (it's equal to the transport capacity, which is typically 10 percent of the maximum amount possible).

LYMPHADENOPATHY: Any disease of the lymph nodes.

LYMPHANGIONS: The one-way lymphatic vessel collector that lies between two heart-shaped valves.

LYMPHATIC AFFERENT VESSELS: Vessels that bring fluid into lymph nodes that contain antigen-presenting cells; antigen, effector, and memory T cells; and regulatory T cells.

LYMPHATIC CAPILLARIES: Overlapping endothelial cells; they are similar to blood capillaries except that they are permeable, allowing lymphatic fluid to enter.

LYMPHATIC COLLECTORS: Also known as lymphatic vessels, they collect and transport lymph.

LYMPHATIC DRAINAGE: A manual technique of soft tissue massage focused on moving lymphatic fluid through the lymphatic system.

LYMPHATIC DRAINS: Another name for lymph nodes.

LYMPHATIC EDUCATION & RESEARCH NETWORK (LE&RN): A lymphatic non-profit with an excellent online source for information about lymphedema and other lymph-related conditions.

LYMPHATIC EFFERENT VESSELS: Vessels that bring fluid out of lymph nodes once it has been been filtered/cleaned.

LYMPHATIC HEALTH CONTINUUM: Refers to a method by which to gauge your lymphatic health using the symptoms of lymph congestion and other comorbidities that play a role in how the lymphatic system functions and influences disease.

LYMPHATIC PRECOLLECTORS: Move lymph into larger lymphatic vessels. They are oriented to absorb fluid. They contain smooth muscle cells and valves to absorb and regulate lymph flow in one direction.

LYMPHATIC TRUNKS: Deeper regions of the lymph network that receive lymphatic fluid from organs, limbs, and areas that act as the final connection between regional lymph nodes and the thoracic duct.

LYMPHEDEMA: A condition in which an accumulation of protein-rich lymphatic fluid builds up in your tissues, causing chronic swelling.

LYMPHOCYTES: White blood cells made in the lymphoid organs that fight off infections, bacteria, and pathogens.

LYMPHOID ORGANS: Small masses of lymph tissue that contain white blood cells to defend against disease in areas where bacteria tends to accumulate, including bone marrow, tonsils and adenoids, thymus, MALT, GALT, spleen, appendix, Peyer's patches, and urinary tract.

LYMPHOTOMES: The areas of the body that drain lymphatic fluid toward regional lymph nodes.

MACROPHAGES: White blood cells that fight off infections and pathogens.

MAMMARY LYMPH NODES: The chain of internal lymph nodes near the sternum and intercostals (rib muscles) that drains a portion of the breasts.

MESENTERIC LYMPH NODES: Lymph nodes in the abdomen that drain the gastrointestinal tract. Part of GALT.

MUCOSA-ASSOCIATED LYMPHOID TISSUE (MALT): Includes the mucous membranes of the skin, eyes, nose, and mouth, nasopharynx, tonsils, salivary glands, thyroid, breast, lungs, respiratory, and urinary and gastrointestinal tracts.

POPLITEAL LYMPH NODES: Lymph nodes located behind the knees.

SAFETY FACTOR: The safety function that responds to an increase in lymph load by increasing its ability to transport lymph.

SUBCLAVIAN VEINS: The right and left lymphatic nodes at the base of the neck that form the juncture with the internal jugular vein to return lymph to the venous system.

SUPERFICIAL LYMPHATIC LAYER: The initial layer of lymph vasculature underneath the skin that carries lymph from the interstitium before it goes to the deeper layers of trunks in the body.

SUPRACLAVICULAR LYMPH NODES: The lymph nodes at the base of the neck above of the clavicle.

THORACIC DUCT: The body's largest lymphatic vessel; it begins in the abdomen and runs up the center of the body, returning lymphatic fluid to the bloodstream near the neck at the left subclavian vein.

TRANSPORT CAPACITY: The maximum amount of lymph that the lymphatic system can handle and transport in a period of time, determined by the capacity of the lymphangions to fill with fluid and their frequency of contractions to propel lymph. In a healthy system it exceeds the lymph load by approximately ten times.

WATERSHEDS: The boundaries separating lymphatic regions/lymphotomes.

ACKNOWLEDGMENTS

I am grateful to many souls for their generosity, support, and commitment, without whom this information might have remained a verbal tradition.

First and foremost are my clients—each and every one of you. Thank you for your faith and trust, and for sharing your journey to health with me.

To my guardian angel, best agent in the business, Dado Derviskadic—you manifested this dream of a book! I am humbled and deeply grateful for your unwavering belief in me, your vision, your laser guidance, and your spiritual counsel. You pushed me to share my work as positively and concisely as possible so that it may serve the highest potential of healing for everyone. I am forever grateful to you for this opportunity and for your irresistible charm and acumen.

Karen Moline—my champion co-writer, cheerleader, organizational guru, and word mistress. I am beyond lucky to have collaborated with you. You worked tirelessly and quickly to help me birth this beast. Your sharp focus and deep investment was a compass among the storms of sentence structure. I value your faith, commitment to excellence, delightful wit, and experienced hand. Thank you from the bottom of my heart for your dedication to this project and to me personally. I'm honored to have done this book with you and I will forever cherish this creation because of your involvement.

Emma Lyddon—illustrator extraordinaire! You are a talented artist of extraordinary measure. In my wildest dreams I couldn't have imagined a better partner to bring the images of the beautiful rivers of lymph into being. You are telepathic and imaginative. You worked every little detail impeccably (and went without sleep for too many days in a row!). You took my childlike scribbles on Post-its and translated visions from my head into artistic treasures. I'm excited for the world to see your talents as I do, full of beauty, and magic. Thank you for gracing these pages with your elegance.

Julie Will—now I know why they refer to you as the Queen of Publishing. You are an editorial genius. Acutely sharp and a perfectionist. Thank you for ensuring that the power and science of lymph is no longer elusive, but instead accessible to the reader. I couldn't have pulled this off without your masterful guidance. I'm deeply grateful to you.

Emma Kupor—a deep, heartfelt thank-you for your insightful edits. You are super-talented and the readers have you (and Julie) to thank for making their experience crystal clear.

Bonni Leon-Berman—thank you for spinning your magic and moving mountains to weave this book together. Your creative genius is evident on every single page. I'm so fortunate to have everyone on my team at Harper Wave. A huge thank you to Karen Rinaldi (visionary leader), Brian Perrin (seasoned marketing prowess), Yelena Nisbit (PR sorceress of excellence and genius), Laura Cole (social maven) and Lynn Anderson (a copy-editor dream), for working hard to bring the best version of this book into as many readers' hands as possible.

Matt—my loving husband, full of integrity and tenderness. You listened to every detail over and over again with patience, investment, thrill, and pride. Marrying you and making a family with you is surely our biggest act of genius. And to our wonderful boys, Isaac and Eddie—your curiosity, humor, warmth, and loving are the stuff dreams are made of. I am so lucky to be your mom. Making chocolate chip cookies together was the propeller to help me get to the finish line. The three of you are glorious humans—you supply me with mountains of encouragement. I'm grateful for you every single day. I love you all so much.

My brother, Steve, my sister-in-law Robin, my niece Jamie, and nephew Ethan—it's never an understatement to say I won the sibling and family lottery. Steve, you have been there for me during the hardest times and best of times. You helped pave a path into a future that Mom would be proud of. I'd be lost in a Guacamole-mobile ditch somewhere without your extreme caring and ESP. KLATM.

My dad, my Poppi—after mom died you took on being the sensitive parent I needed. You showed me how to create boundaries and foster self-worth. You instilled a sense of adventure and wanderlust and reminded me time and time again that I was capable of anything I set my mind to. Thank you for always supporting me as best you could. You're truly an ox. And, it's a tie . . .

My mom, Edie, who was ahead of her time. She spread a trail of graceful empowerment in her life and in her passing as well. With twinkling laughter in her eyes, a strong sense of self-worth and compassion, her spirit is still a guiding light within me, and her imprint is more powerful now than ever before.

To my loving and supportive family, I am who I am because of you. My beautiful sister Renee Levitt, my humorous brother Michael Levitt and his family, Gloria, Sheila, Priscila, and Matthew—I love you all dearly! My jackpot supportive in-laws Adele and Bruce Gainsley, and Jessie, Ben, and Joaquin Rivera—*mi familia, te amo mucho!* Uncle Eddie, Aunt Sylvia, Uncle Jules, Kristine, Eileen, Uncle Norm, Aunt Lois, Aunt Rheva, Uncle Gary, Uncle Hank, and Carol. To my very special cousin Ronna Evans, who introduced me to the spirit world. And to my dozens of cousins who always lead with their heart.

To the best friends a girl could have—you have all contributed to the existence of this book in countless ways with your laughter, epic wine collection, homemade dolmas and chocolates, international adventures, social justice work, lymphatic workshop hosting, imperative counsel, and deep friendship. Bust (Jen), Mikey and Daniella Lippman; Hilary

Webb; Kat Jarvis and Ross MacKenzie; Rebecca Starr; Libby Marsh; Rhonda, Todd, Drea, Ezra, and Ari Buchman; Megan and David Dobkin; Tiffany Siart and Jango Sircus; Rochelle Rose and Tim Merrill; Jefferey MacIntyre and Haigaz Farajian; Wendy and Jon Mantell.

Thank you to these helpful angels—Ashlee Margolis, Larry David, Freida Pinto, Jenni Kayne, Selma Blair, Candace Nelson, Susanna Felleman, Kimberly and Michael Muller, Laura Ziskin, Julia Barry, Dr. Gottfried Konecny, Rachel Frankenthal, Rory Green, Rachel Krupa, John and Dana Kibler, Seane Corn, Allison Oswald, Pam Daughlin, and Jess Zanotti.

Evelyn—the first to support my career as lymphatic therapist before anyone knew what that meant.

Patricia Wiltse—my initial lymphatic teacher, whose golden hands and commitment to the integrity of lymphatic drainage lineage showed me how to love my lymph and the bedrock of science that it's built on. Pat taught me unconditional acceptance and how to allow energy to flow through my hands to be a catalyst for self-healing.

My lymphatic colleagues and trailblazers—Maureen McBeth, Steve Norton, Joachim Zuther, Gunter Klose, William Rippicci, The Lymphatic Education & Research Network (LE&RN), Dr. Stanley Rockson, Kathy Bates, Dr. Ketan Patel, The National Lymphedema Network (NLN), Drs. Emil and Estrid Vodder, and Professors Michael and Ethel Foeldi—you maintain the highest standards of lymphatic knowledge. The world is lucky to have you in its midst.

Dr. H.J.A. Gochette, DC, and Carol White, MN, NP, at New Millennium Institute of Wellness. Thank you for taking such wonderful care of me and my family physically, spiritually, and holistically with your alchemy.

Finally, many thanks to every single one of you who has picked up this book and is curious about the powers of lymph!

INDEX

Herophilos, 27

Hippocampus, 201, 225

Hippocrates, 26–27, *30*

Holistic remedies, xv. *See also* Self-
care routines

Hormone imbalances, 33. *See also*
Menopause; Premenstrual
syndrome symptom relief

Hydration, 73, 278, 280

Hyperthyroidism, 71

Hypotension, 71

Iliac nodes, 200

Immune system, 5–6, 23–25, 38,
41–42, 46, 56, 123, 270

Immunoglobin A, 24–25

Inflammation
acute, 40, 41, 84, 214
anti-inflammatory foods, 63,
272–75, *273*
anti-inflammatory herbs, 83, 278,
279
chronic, 26, 34, 39, 41–42
lymphatic congestion and, xvi,
xviii, 26, 38
of the skin, 33, 42, 129–31. *See
also* Acne
symptoms of, 41
use of term, 38

Infrared biomats, 51, 300

Infrared lasers, 301

Infrared saunas, 301

Inguinal lymph nodes, 264, 319

Innate immunity, 25

Insomnia. *See* Sleep

Institute of Conscious BodyWork,
xv–xvi

Internal landscape, 148–88
calm anxiety, 148–56
energy and mental clarity,
157–65
good sleep, 181–88
hangover remedy, 165–72
heart and lung opener, 173–80

Interstitial fluid, 6, 7, 12, 319

Irritable bowel syndrome (IBS), 42,
277

Isolated lymphoid follicles (ILFs),
23, 24

Jade rolling, 225, 290

J-stroke, 76, *76*

Kapha, *55*

Keto diet, 270–71

Ketosis, 271

Kidney disease, 33

Kidneys, 7, 123

Kinesiology (kinesio) taping,
308